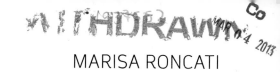

MARISA RONCATI

GET SHARP

NONSURGICAL PERIODONTAL INSTRUMENT SHARPENING

Q_e

Milan | Berlin | Chicago | Tokyo | Barcelona | Istanbul | London | Moscow | New Delhi | Paris | Peking | Prague | Sân Paulo | Seoul | Warsaw

© 2011 Quintessenza Edizioni
Via Ciro Menotti, 65 - 20017 Rho, Milano (Italy)
Tel. +39 02 93180821 - Fax +39 02 93186159
e-mail: info@quintessenzaedizioni.it
www.quintessenzaedizioni.it

Project manager: Dr. Stefano Sicura
Graphic design: Borgo Creativo
Illustrations: Elisa Botton

Printed in Italy

ISBN 978-88-7492-153-9

To my father Luciano Roncati,

A simply extraordinary person because of his intelligence, manual ability, creativity, precision, and competence in several fields.
A man with a continuously and inexhaustibly active brain, capable of truly brilliant solutions, full of energy and sincere enthusiasm for multiple interests, always happy to offer his precious help with good humor, and, above all, a man whose biological age does not coincide with the chronological one!

ACKNOWLEDGMENTS

From the bottom of my heart, I would like to thank all the staff at the Parma Benfenati dental office, particularly Barbara Bertasi, Barbara Oghittu, and Irene Carlino for their valuable photo documentation, Dario Giordano for software support and Elisa Botton for the text illustrations.

MARISA RONCATI

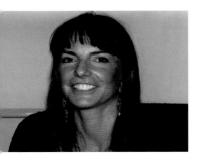

Degree in Classical Literature.

Registered Dental Hygienist RDH at Forsyth School for Dental Hygienists, Boston (U.S.A.).

Degree in Dentistry and Dental Prosthesis (DDS) at the University of Ferrara, Italy.

Assistant Professor at School of Dental Hygiene at the University of Bologna (1991 to 2002) and the University of Ferrara (2002 to 2006).

Assistant Professor at School of Dental Hygiene at the Università Politecnica delle Marche (2008 to present) Chairman: Professor A. Putignano.

Lecturer in didactic Module: "Postprosthetic Follow-up and Professional Hygiene" at the Master of Prosthesis and Implantology with Advanced Technologies at the University of Bologna, DEAN Professor Roberto Scotti.

Lecturer in Module 7: Laser in Periodontics and Implantology of the European Master Degree on Oral Laser's Applications, Chairman: Prof. U. Romeo, La Sapienza, University of Rome.

Lecturer in didactic Module at the Master in Implantology, University of Padova dean: Professor Antonio Favero.

FOREWORD

I became acquainted with Marisa many years ago at important research congresses around the world. Attendance at these events is proof of her continuous efforts to study and update her knowledge base in a constant search for quality. Nevertheless, my consideration for her increased further when I again met her, this time in the role of spokeswoman, and I saw her ability to transmit knowledge and enthusiasm into the dental profession, which has developed to become the fundamental presupposition for the success of any therapy.

When I became Chairman of the School for Dental Hygienists at my University, her skills compelled me to ask her to use her experience in the service of our students.

I have followed every step in the realization of this book, to which Marisa has dedicated much of her time. Because of this dedication, she has produced a text on a subject that I consider to be fundamental: the sharpening of nonsurgical periodontal instruments.

In this well-illustrated book, the reader will find techniques and useful suggestions to achieve correct instrument sharpening.

I believe that this text is intended for whomever wishes to learn, investigate, and improve their knowledge of this subject, which I consider to be fundamental to treatment planning.

Professor Angelo Putignano
Chairman, School for Dental Hygienists
Università Politecnica delle Marche - Ancona, Italy

PREFACE

Learning how to sharpen instruments correctly is not a simple task.
I discovered that even I was making mistakes when sharpening nonsurgical peri-odontal instruments, although I had diligently studied the principles and rules of sharpening techniques. Moreover, in teaching students and colleagues how to sharpen their own instruments, I still encountered difficulties.
I feel that learning the techniques for sharpening and their application in daily practice must be supported by illustrations and schematics that can simplify the student's understanding of the task.
I have tried to be very didactic and as clear as possible in my explanations, re-ducing the sharpening angles that must be memorized to three: 20, 40, and 45 degrees.
Careful attention on the part of the student will avoid mistakes that are quite fre-quent in clinical practice, as detailed in Chapter 5. Sharpening mistakes modify the characteristics of the instrument, jeopardizing its efficiency and negatively in-fluencing tissue healing.
Time dedicated to sharpening is always a good investment! Root instrumenta-tion with unsharpened instruments is difficult and tiring but, above all, is associ-ated with inadequate and unsafe treatment. Moreover, an unsharpened instru-ment can burnish the deposits of calculus, removing the calculus only partially, and consequently leading to incomplete healing. Therefore, sharpening is a daily necessity, and it must be well-learned to obtain the maximum advantage from instrumentation.
Sharpening is a necessary maintenance that extends the life of all instruments and has a significant economic impact.

Marisa Roncati

CONTENTS

GET SHARP
NONSURGICAL PERIODONTAL INSTRUMENT SHARPENING

01

11   WHY SHARPEN?
12   The purpose of instrument sharpening
15   Advantages of a well sharpened instrument
16   Disadvantages of a dull instrument
18   Goals of instrument sharpening
20   Rationale for manual sharpening

02

21   WHEN SHARPEN?
24   Maintaining sterility while sharpening during treatment

03

27   SHARPENING MATERIALS
28   Armamentarium
30   Sharpening stones
     30   Origin
     32   Shape
     33   Degree of abrasiveness
37   Lubricants
38   Tool for evaluating sharpness

04

39   ANATOMY OF NONSURGICAL PERIODONTAL INSTRUMENTS
40   General features of periodontal instruments
     41   Handle
     44   Shank
     47   Working end
58   Standard instruments and rigid instruments
59   Classification of nonsurgical periodontal instruments
     59   Sickle scalers
     61   Curets
     62   Files
     63   Hoes
     64   Universal instruments
     68   Area-specific instruments
72   The minimal nonsurgical periodontal instrument kit

05 73 SHARPENING ERRORS
74 Do not sharpen every instrument using the same angle between stone and handle
84 Do not forget sharpening the tip of the curet, whether universal or area-specific
89 Do not sharpen the instrument frontal surface

06 91 CORRECT SHARPENING TECHNIQUES
94 Sharpening methods
94 Stationary stone/moving instrument technique
98 Stationary instrument/moving stone technique
100 Sharpening the universal curet
105 Sharpening the area-specific curet
111 Sharpening the scaler

118 REFERENCES

119 VERIFICATION QUESTIONS AND ANSWERS

WHY SHARPEN?

01

GET SHARP
NONSURGICAL PERIODONTAL INSTRUMENT SHARPENING

THE PURPOSE OF INSTRUMENT SHARPENING

A well-sharpened instrument DETERMINES a more effective periodontal instrumentation. Conversely, a blunt instrument is likely
to leave residual calculus, which in turn not only undermine the
efficiency of the instrumentation, but also can jeopardize the
healing of the site.

All new instruments generally have a very sharp blade, but frequent
use soon dulls the cutting edge, consequently reducing efficiency of
instrumentation.

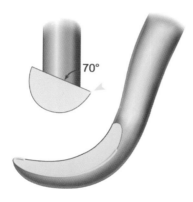

Sharp area specific Curet

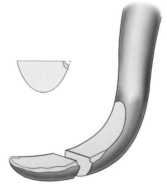

Blunt area specific Curet

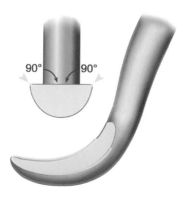

Sharp Universal Curet

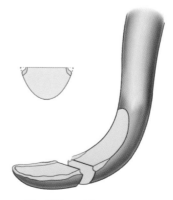

Blunt Universal Curet

In selecting the instruments, we look at the handle that has to facilitate a good grip, we control the shank, more or less angled, then search for a blade, preferably miniaturized, especially for advanced instrumentation in deep pockets.

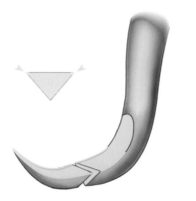 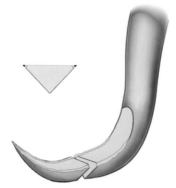

Sharp sickle scaler   **Blunt** sickle scaler

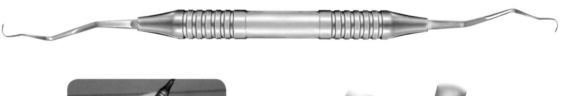

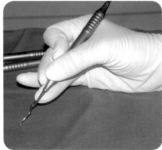 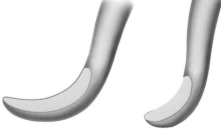

During treatment, the operator must constantly confirm the efficiency of the instrument's cutting edge in removing calculus deposits.

Very often, instruments become prematurely useless because of inadequate sharpening technique, sooner than as a result of regular wear.

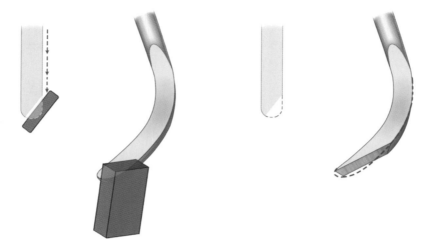

These figures show how the original profile of an instrument can be distorted by an incorrectly positioned sharpening stone.

The most important quality of a periodontal instrument is its degree of sharpness. Learning how to sharpen instruments correctly is not effortless. Some basic information and a good deal of patience are required to learn the exact technique.

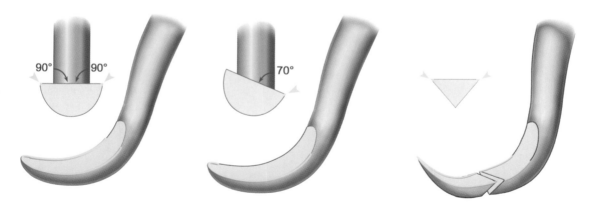

The key purposes of dental instrument sharpening are twofold:
1. to restore a sharp cutting edge
2. to preserve the original shape of the instrument

ADVANTAGES:
A WELL SHARPENED INSTRUMENT

1. better control by the clinician, improving dexterity and accuracy
2. precludes unnecessary trauma to gingival tissue, which minimizes patient discomfort (prevents accidental trauma to the mucous tissue, which means less discomfort for the patient)
3. does not have to be grasped as tightly as a dull on, reducing hand fatigue
4. improves tactile sensitivity during instrumentation
5. allows the clinician to hook the interface between root surface and deposits to remove them, with less likelihood of burnishing rather than removing the calculus[15]

CORRECT NONSURGICAL PERIODONTAL INSTRUMENTATION TECHNIQUE

The instrument is inserted subgingivally until it reaches the most apical extension of the calcified deposit, which is engaged and completely removed.

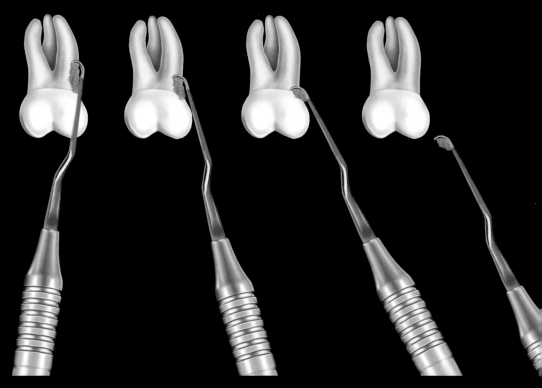

6. decreases the risk of nicking, scratching or creating grooves on the root surface
7. reduces the numbers of needed working strokes, shortening the working time
8. is less fatiguing for the clinician (Reduces operator fatigue)
9. performs non surgical periodontal instrumentation more effectively
10. allows a more accurate treatment and improves the quality of results[1]

In summary: a sharp instrument does **promote** efficiency of periodontal instrumentation.

DISADVANTAGES OF A DULL INSTRUMENT

• the operator may lose control of the instrument
• the patient's comfort level is decreased, and he may be exposed to the risk of tissue trauma
• working time is increased. Nonsurgical periodontal treatment with dull instruments requires more time; it has been shown that the working time with unsharpened instruments is about two-thirds longer[2-4]
• the operator tends to compensate for instrument inefficiency by applying increased pressure to the tooth surface
• the operator is subjected to greater fatigue

Most importantly:
• the calculus may be burnished, when only its superficial layer is removed
• the remaining calculus substrate can be difficult to detect, even with a periodontal explorer
• the presence of residual calculus can jeopardize ideal healing of the instrumented site

INCORRECT NONSURGICAL PERIODONTAL INSTRUMENTATION TECHNIQUE

Incorrect instrumentation will not fully remove the calculus deposit but will instead burnish it. Burnishing is defined as the removal of only the superficial part of the calculus, leaving some residual calcified deposits on the root surface after instrumentation is complete. The cause of burnishing is incorrect scaling technique. Instead of moving the handle away from the root surface, in the correct working stroke, the instrument moves in a coronal direction, causing the deposit to be burnished.

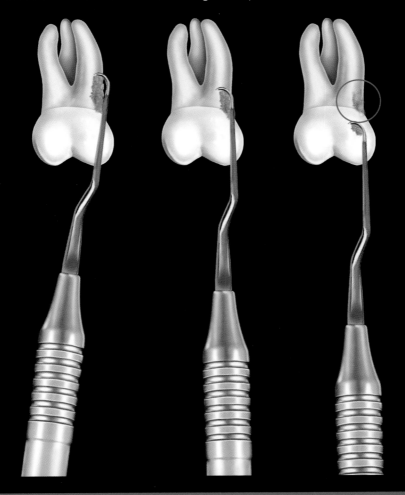

In summary: an dull instrument **jeopardizes** the efficiency of instrumentation because it produces residual calculus,[5-7] which in turn can impair ideal healing.

GOALS OF INSTRUMENT SHARPENING

1 • TO PRESERVE THE ORIGINAL SHAPE OF THE INSTRUMENT

Sharpening curets, it is crucial to pay special attention at the tip, which must maintain its characteristic roundness.

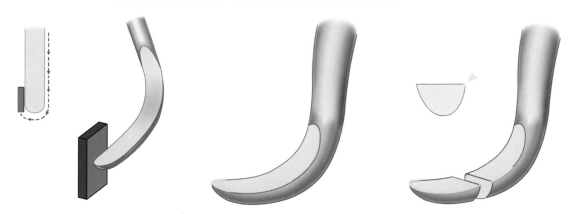

The figure on the left shows the path of the sharpening stone as it uniformly abrades the lateral surface of the instrument. The tip must also be sharpened so that the instrument dimensions are reduced proportionally.

2 • TO RESTORE A WELL-SHARPENED CUTTING EDGE

The cutting edge has a length, but no thickness.

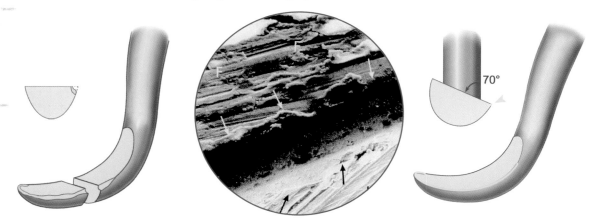

The figure on the left shows that loss of sharpness has created a third surface between the facial and lateral surfaces of the instrument, as a result of dulling. The scanning electron microscope

(SEM) image at original magnification x300 shows a third surface between the lateral surface (black arrows) and facial surface (white arrows) of the instrument.[2,8,9] Conversely, the figure on the right shows a well-sharpened cutting edge associated with a single dimension, its length.

3 • TO AVOID EXCESSIVE WEAR OF THE INSTRUMENT

Be careful to correctly place the stone. Focus on the right angle between stone and frontal surface, in order to preserve the original 70° angle between the frontal and the lateral surface of the instrument.

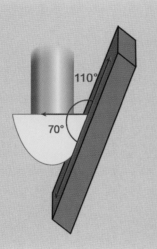

YES

Correct angle: the stone is properly positioned against the lateral surface, maintaining the internal angle of 70 degrees.

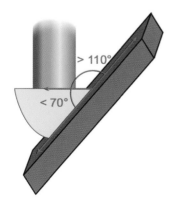

NO

Incorrect angle: the stone is too angled, creating an internal angle lower than 70 degrees. Consequently, the cutting edge will work efficiently at first but it dulls very quickly, and after few working strokes, the instrument requires further sharpening.

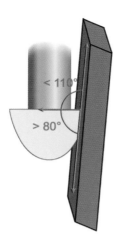

NO

Incorrect angle: the stone is not sufficiently angled, creating an internal angle greater than 70 degrees. Consequently, the working edge turns out to be too bulky, and it will be difficult to adjust the blade to the tooth.

RATIONALE FOR MANUAL SHARPENING

Manual sharpening is the method of choice for refreshing instrument blades while working. Moreover, the sharp edge is reduced more gradually compare to the aggressiveness of the cut made with mounted stone[1], given the same manual expertise in both methods.
Even with proper training, manual sharpening is more consistent than power-driven sharpening, which can very likely remove excessive metal. Frictional heat may also affect the temper of the steel.[1]
Sharpening is therefore a daily need, and the technique must be properly learned so that the operator uses his or her time in the most profitable way.

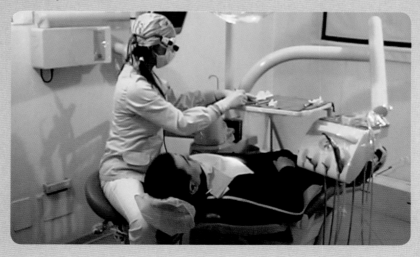

WHEN SHARPEN? MAINTAINING STERILITY WHILE SHARPENING DURING TREATMENT

02

GET SHARP
NONSURGICAL PERIODONTAL INSTRUMENT SHARPENING

Instruments must be sharpened at the first sign of dullness, of their in-effective debridement, when the instrument stops emitting the typical scraping sound during instrumentation.

It is easier for the operator to sharpen an instrument whose cutting edge has just lost its sharpness than to wait until the instrument is grossly dull and very inefficient.

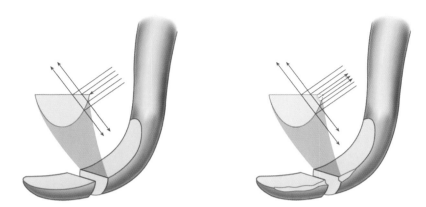

When the instrument has a blunt edging, a third, but pernicious surface is been created between the frontal surface and the lateral one, this new surface, no more cutting, will reflect the light, under a source of illumination.

Sharpen at the first sign of dullness during periodontal instrumentation. Don't let your instruments become totally ineffective. It will be easier on clinician and better for long term instruments maintenance care.

First of all the time spent sharpening is gained back in efficiency and in effective outcomes.

Lastly recontouring grossly dulled instruments into a sharp blade is arduous to achieve.

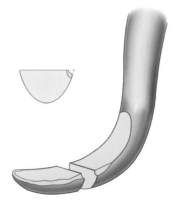 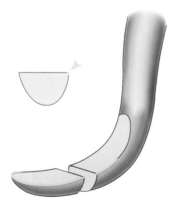 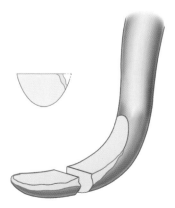

Sometimes, the operator feels that he or she lacks the time for sharpening and continues to work in a difficult and tiring way with inadequate results because he or she does not want to "waste time". In doing so, the operator risks harming the patient; the calculus deposits are burnished, preventing complete healing of the instrumented site.

First of all the time spent sharpening is gained back in efficiency and in effective outcomes.

Lastly recontouring grossly dulled instruments into a sharp blade is arduous to achieve.[1,2,10]

If an dental auxiliary is well instructed in sharpening, it is recommended to perform it on sterile instruments, so to prevent accidental puncture, and then to autoclave sharpened instruments again, prior to chair-side use.

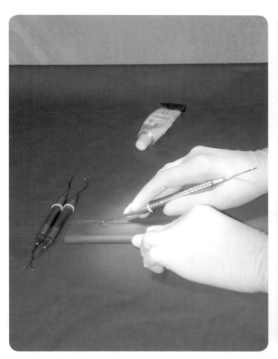
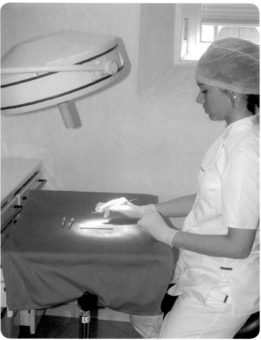

Contrary to earlier belief, sterilization does not modify the degree of sharpness of a good-quality instrument. Viceversa, in case the operator who sharpens the instruments will also be using them, it is convenient to sharpen them during clinical activity. In such a case it is mandatory to have a high regard for asepsy.

MAINTAINING STERILITY WHILE SHARPENING DURING TREATMENT

If the person who sharpens the instruments will also be using them, it is better to sharpen them during treatment. There may be a sterile stone ready for use on the dental hygiene tray. The stone must be prepared and already lubricated before beginning the clinical session.

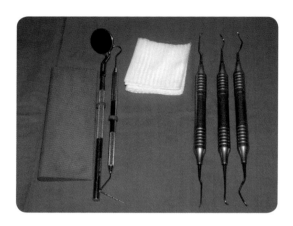

Otherwise The operator may feel the need to sharpen the instruments during the course of treatment without having planned it early, because a cutting edge can become dull after 40 to 60 working strokes, in which case you must respect the asepsis. To do this, the operator turns to an assistant with the following request:
"Would you please bring me a sharpening stone and some lubricant? Thank you!"

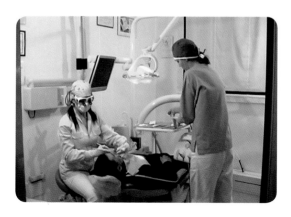

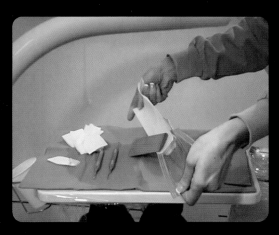

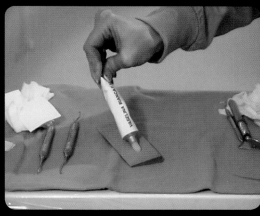

The assistant brings a sterilized stone to the operatory and, with bare hands, opens the envelope to drop the stone onto the tray.

The assistant puts the sterilized envelope aside and, still with bare hands, unscrews the cap of the lubricant and dispenses some onto the stone, without contaminating it.

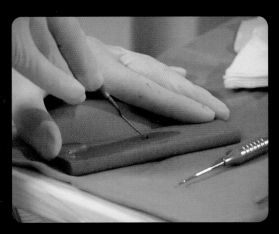

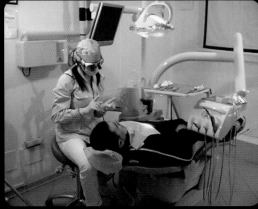

The operator then distributes petroleum jelly over the stone and begins to sharpen the instruments.

In addition to maintaining sterility, it is important for the operator to explain this procedure to the patient, saying for example: **"Now I am sharpening the instruments to make them more effective, certainly not to make them more aggressive."**

Often, a few sharpening strokes are sufficient to renew the cutting edge of the instruments. In the course of sharpening, the sludge, or metal particles removed during grinding remain attached to the edge of the instrument. The wire edge created during this procedure can be removed with gauze moistened with disinfectant.

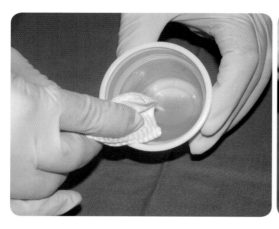
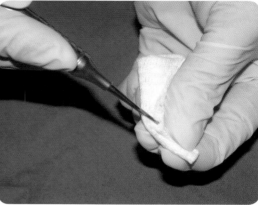

It is then possible to resume instrumentation in a different area of the oral cavity as needed, efficiently removing the calculus deposits without burnishing them.

Time dedicated to sharpening is surely a good investment.

Do not postpone sharpening during the course of treatment because the instruments could become so grossly dull that restoring a well-sharpened cutting edge could be very difficult to achieve.

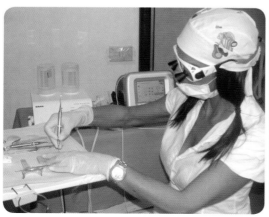
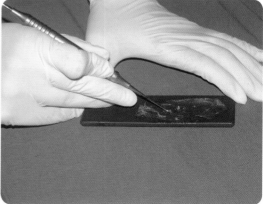

SHARPENING MATERIALS

03

GET SHARP
NONSURGICAL PERIODONTAL INSTRUMENT SHARPENING

ARMAMENTARIUM

All stones are adequate for sharpening; the sharpening technique is more important than the type of the stone selected. Therefore, it is advisable to use stones that are readily available in the clinical equipment and to follow the sharpening techniques described in this text. If it is necessary or desirable to buy a new sharpening stone, the India stone, either rectangular and flat or wedge-shaped, is recommended.

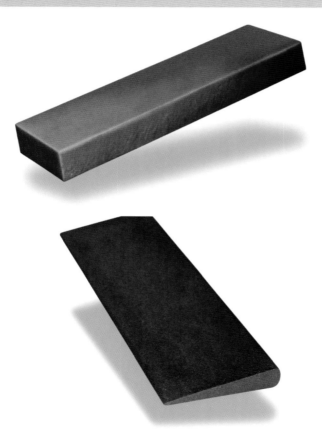

Sharpening is a procedure requiring high precision and can be made easier by strong illumination and a magnification system. Even a simple magnifying lens will improve the operator's visualization of the cutting edge to be sharpened (the dull cutting edge presents a rounded, shiny surface which reflects light). The magnifying lens can help the operator to determine if sharpening is needed, to view the worn edge, and, most importantly, to study the original shape of the instrument so that it is not modified by incorrect sharpening.

Essential materials for sharpening:

- magnifying lens or magnifying loops
- sharpening stone
- lubricant
- acrylic testing stick
- gauze
- detergent solution such as orange solvent

...**and obviously**, the instruments to be sharpened.

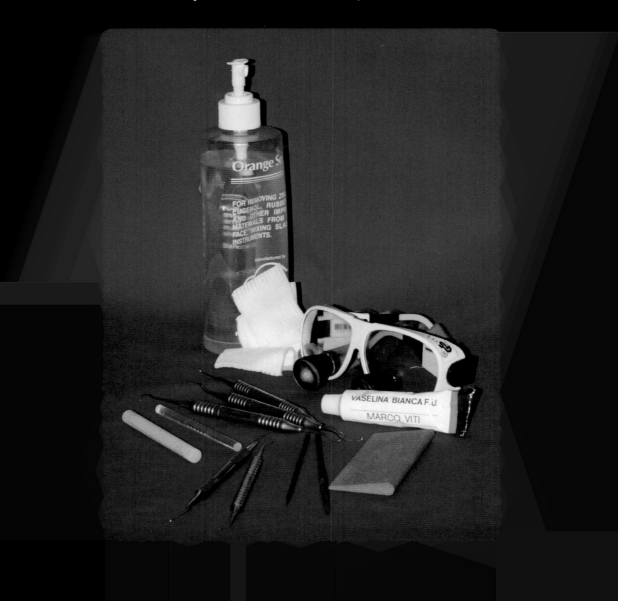

SHARPENING STONES

An India stone, either rectangular and flat or wedge-shaped, is preferred.

Sharpening stones can be classified by reason of several characteristics:
1 • origin,
2 • shape,
3 • degree of abrasiveness.

1 • ORIGIN

A) **Natural abrasive stones**, quarried from mineral deposits.

India stones: this stone is the author's first choice. It is available in only one degree of abrasiveness.

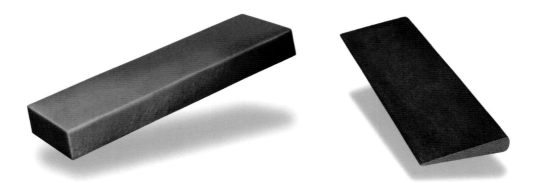

Arkansas stones: these stones are less preferable because they are available in various degrees of abrasiveness, some of which are only slightly abrasive and therefore not suitable for grossly dull instruments. They are useful for refining a sharpened edge and may be adequate for instruments requiring minimal sharpening; they may also be used for a more prudent, conservative sharpening technique.

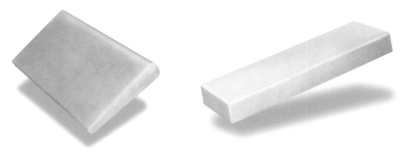

B) Synthetic and man-made abrasive industrial-type stones.

These stones are composed of nonmetallic hard substances such as diamond particles, aluminum oxide, tungsten or silicon carbide.

Because these are generally larger and coarser than particles of theArkansas stone,[1] synthetic stones may be too abrasive for manual sharpening. They may be utilized in **mechanical sharpening devices** and power-driven sharpening equipment.

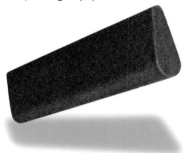

Ceramic stones: of industrial origin; these stones have a very fine grain and therefore are not abrasive enough for sharpening very dull instruments.

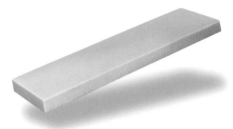

Ceramic stones may be mounted on a metal mandrel[11] and are used in a motor driven handpiece.

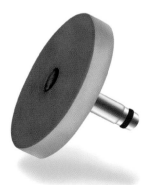
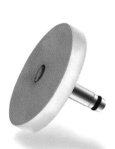
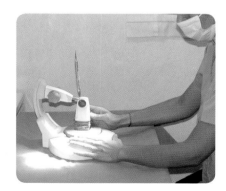

2 • SHAPE

Flat rectangular stones

Use of this stone is suggested; with its squared angles, it simplifies the estimation of the correct angle between the instrument and the stone, as compared to the wedge-shaped stone.

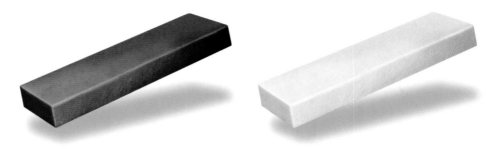

Wedge-shaped rectangular stones

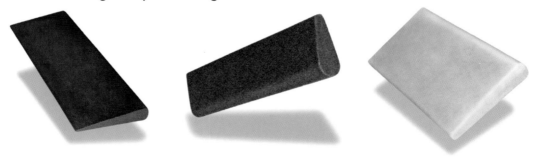

Cylindrical stones, straight or pointed

The cylindrical stone is indicated only as a refining, postsharpening instrument for the elimination of metallic "wire edge". It is not essential but can be useful.

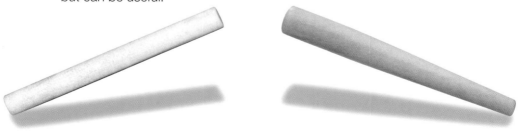

3 • DEGREE OF ABRASIVENESS

The surface of the stone consists of crystalline particles, abrasive elements that sharpen the instrument.[1,12] The dimensions of such particles influence the degree of abrasiveness: particles of smaller dimension are present in fine-grain stones and **determine** a slower sharpening procedure.

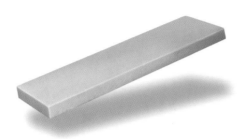

Fine grain
Arkansas and ceramic stones
Use of these stones is not strongly suggested. Preferably, they are indicated for instruments that are slightly dull or for refinement of sharpening.

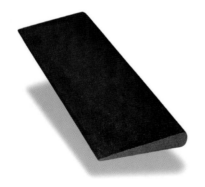

Medium grain
India stones
This stone is preferred because it is useful for routine sharpening. Moreover, it is indicated for re-creating the cutting profile of instruments that are badly worn or require extensive reshaping after incorrect sharpening.

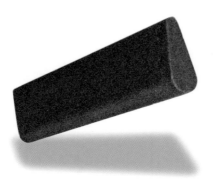

Coarse grain
Stones of industrial origin
Stones composed of carborundum or diamond hone are often too abrasive for routine instrument sharpening. Moreover, if used incorrectly, they can easily modify the original design of the instrument.

COMPARISON TABLE OF THE SHARPENING STONES

	Type of stone	Origin	Lubricant	Grain	Indications for use	Shape
FIRST PREFERENCE	India	Natural	Petroleum jelly	Medium	Routine sharpening	Rectangular and flat or wedge-shaped
SECOND PREFERENCE	Arkansas	Natural	Petroleum jelly	Fine	Refinement after routine sharpening; sharpening of well-maintained instruments	Rectangular and flat or wedge-shaped; cylindrical and pointed or straight
NOT RECOMMENDED	Ceramic	Industrial	Water	Fine	Refinement after routine sharpening; sharpening of well-maintained instruments. Can be mounted on a metal mandrel for motor-driven sharpening devices	Rectangular and flat
NOT RECOMMENDED	Carborundum	Industrial	Water	Coarse	Sharpening excessively dull cutting edges; should be used by skilled operators only	Wedge-shaped
NOT RECOMMENDED	Diamond	Industrial	Water	Coarse	Sharpening excessively dull cutting edges and instrument requiring an extreme degree of contouring; should be used by skilled operators only	Rectangular and flat

There is a specific stone for sharpening **Hirschfeld periodontal files** called **file sharpener**; it is available in flat and triangular versions. Its dimensions range from 10 to 14 cm.

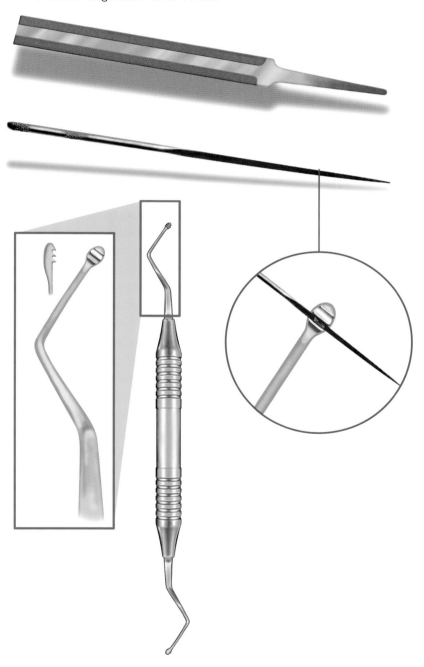

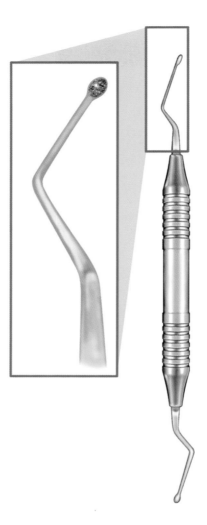

If the operator uses periodontal files, such as the Hirschfeld periodontal files, the file sharpener must also be purchased. An exception is the **Roncati File**, which has a modified diamond-coated surface and does not need to be sharpened.

LUBRICANTS

The stone must be always be lubricated before sharpening. India and Arkansas stones should be lubricated with white petroleum jelly (or mineral oil).

Why it is necessary to lubricate the stone?

- to allow the instrument blade to glide smoothly over the stone
- to minimize clogging of the pores of the stone by metallic particles removed during sharpening
- to prevent excessive wear of the instrument
- to reduce heat produced by friction

Instruments should never be sharpened on a dry stone because the continuous friction between the stone and the instrument creates heat, which can cause the metal to become more fragile.[1,7,12,13]

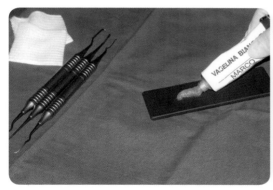
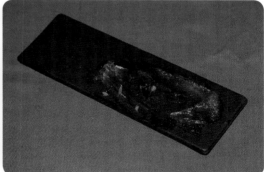
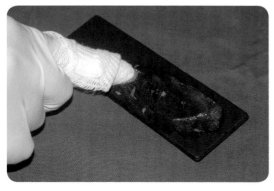

The lubricant, either mineral oil or, preferably, petroleum jelly, is uniformly distributed on the stone with a gauze.

TOOL FOR EVALUATING SHARPNESS

Plastic (acrylic) testing stick

A plastic or acrylic testing stick (1/4 inch rod, 3 inches long) is used to evaluate the cutting efficiency and degree of sharpening achieved after the sharpening procedure. This instrument can be sterilized in autoclave.

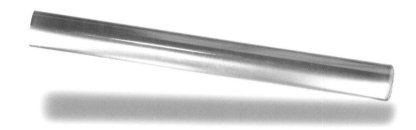

ANATOMY OF NONSURGICAL PERIODONTAL INSTRUMENTS

04

GET SHARP
NONSURGICAL PERIODONTAL INSTRUMENT SHARPENING

GENERAL FEATURES
OF PERIODONTAL INSTRUMENTS

All instruments present:

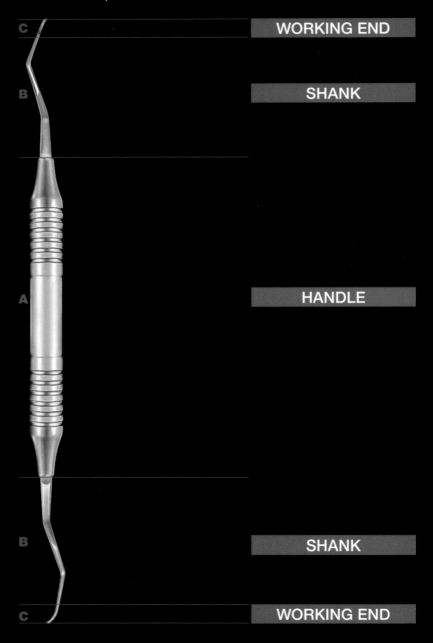

C — WORKING END

B — SHANK

A — HANDLE

B — SHANK

C — WORKING END

A • HANDLE

Handle styles and materials vary widely.

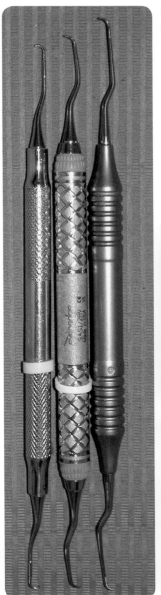

Instrument handles with certain features are recommended:

- a hollow handle will improve the operator's tactile sense, minimizing effort
- a handle that is not overly slender will avoid muscle cramps and prevent Carpal Tunnel Syndrome
- a textured handle will improve the operator's grasp and reduce finger fatigue

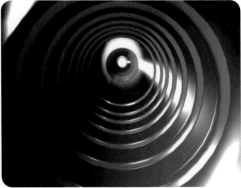

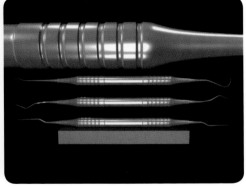

Shape and size of the handle can facilitate operator dexterity and also prevent work-related disorders; but for this specific purpose is much more significant the instrument grasp in addition to the technique adopted by the operator during instrumentation, over the type of instrument selected.

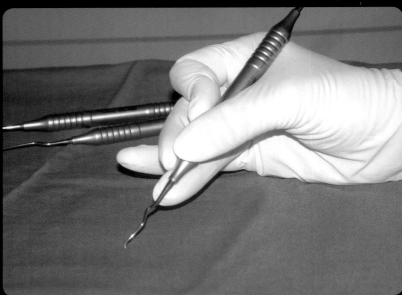

In case the instruments available for use lack the suggested characteristics, ie: the instruments have smooth, thin handles, it is still possible to avoid muscular fatigue as well as prevent Carpal Tunnel Syndrome. The operator should simply alternate a strong grasp with a delicate one, such as the light grasp indicated for probing calculus deposits before their removal.

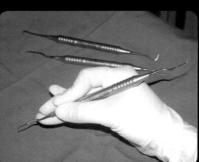
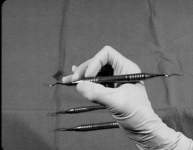

Another useful suggestion for preventing muscular fatigue is to stretch fingers and hands periodically during the working day, for istance while the patient is rinsing or otherwise occupied.

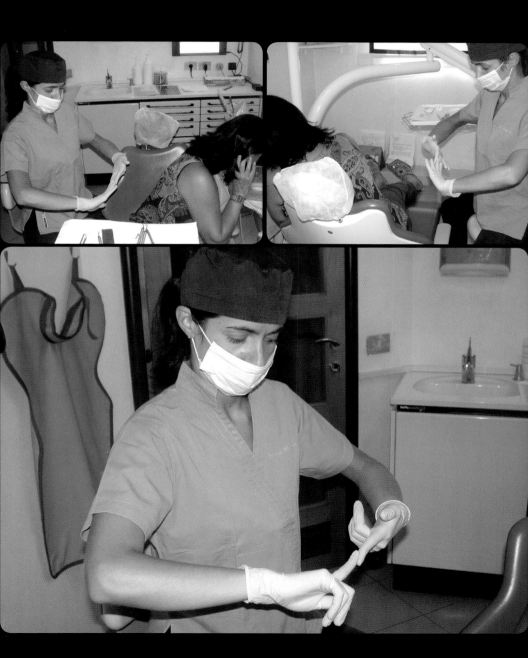

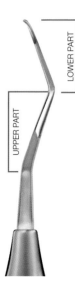

LOWER PART

UPPER PART

B • SHANK

The shank extends from the handle neck up to the working end. We distinguish a lower and an upper part of the shank.

- The lower part of the shank is closer to the working end and extends from the end of the blade to the first curve of the shank. It is extremely important to know the anatomy of the shank to distinguish whether a curet is Universal or Area Specific.
- The upper part of the shank extends from its first curve to the handle.

In this text we focus on the angle created between the lower part of the shank and the stone to indicate the sharpening angle for different kinds of instruments.

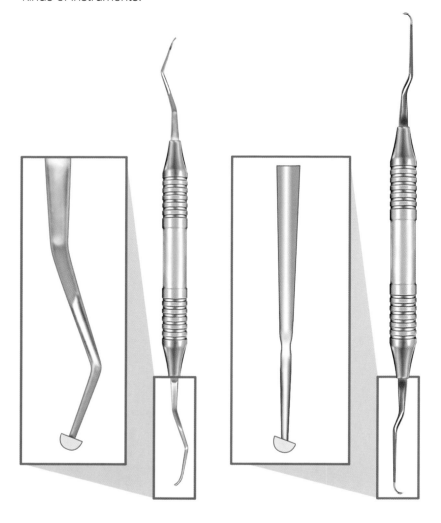

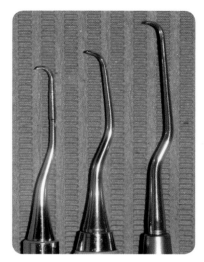

In some curet, such as the Mini and After Five* Curets, terminal shank is redesigned to be 3 mm longer than the corresponding standard-shank Gracey Curets. This segment is elongated by 3 mm, compared with the corresponding instrument in the standard version, to access root surfaces and 5 mm or deeper periodontal pockets. Instruments with a longer stalk are preferable, even though shank length is not the most significant characteristic of these instruments, to facilitate an effective periodontal instrumentation. The reduced size of the blade actually influences the result more so than the shank dimension. To instrument narrow and deep periodontal pockets I do prefer miniaturized instruments (Mini. Curets).

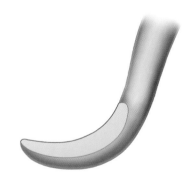

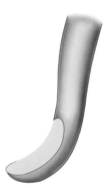

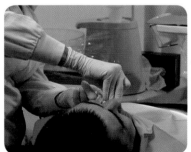

I also personally support the use of extra oral fulcrum or **not dominant** hand reinforcement that can possibly facilitate deep periodontal instrumentation, compensating for the standard size shank type of instruments. Thinned blade are chosen to ease gingival insertion and reduce tissue distention. When available, rigid or extra rigid design curet should be chosen for greater strength and for aggressive instrumentation, when needed.

Different types of instruments can exhibit a **straight** or an **angled shanks**.

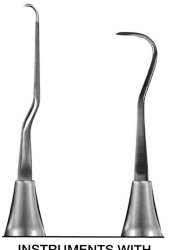 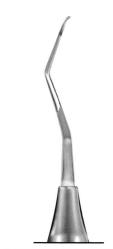

**INSTRUMENTS WITH
A STRAIGHT SHANK**

**INSTRUMENT WITH
AN ANGULATED SHANK**

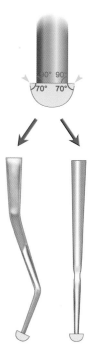

universal curets

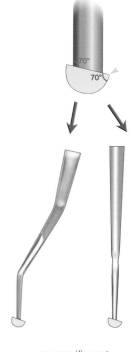

area-specific curets

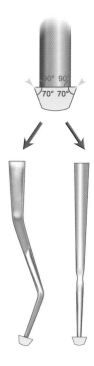

sickle scalers

C • WORKING END

The working end is the terminal segment of the instrument. Area-specific instruments have only one cutting edge. The cutting edge is located on the lower edge of the facial surface. The face of the blade is "off-set", at an angle of approximately 70 degrees, in relation to the lower shank.

AREA-SPECIFIC INSTRUMENT

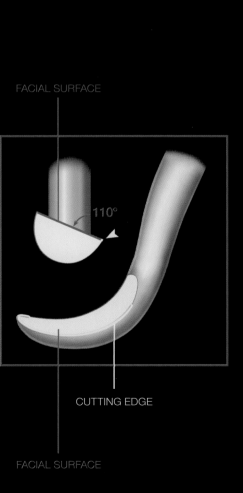

FACIAL SURFACE

110°

CUTTING EDGE

FACIAL SURFACE

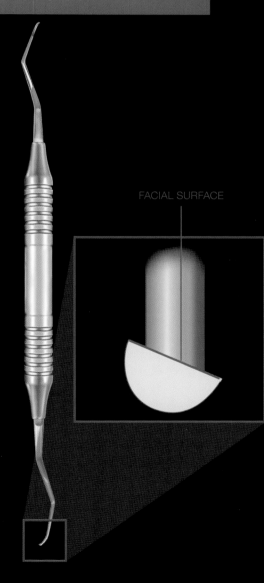

FACIAL SURFACE

Universal instruments have two cutting edges which meet to form a rounded tip or toe. These cutting edge are created by the junction of the flat face and the curved sides or lateral surfaces of the working end. The lateral surfaces, in turn, extend from each cutting edge and converge to shape the convex back of the blade. The face of the blade is perpendicular, at a 90-degree angle in relation to the lower shank.

UNIVERSAL INSTRUMENT

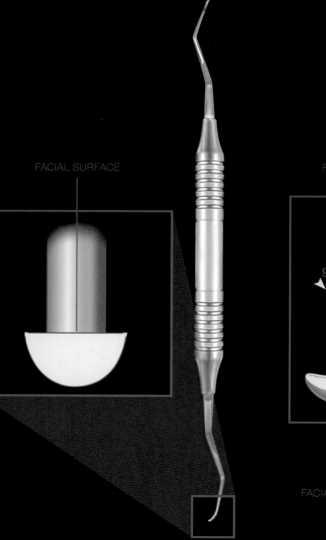

FACIAL SURFACE

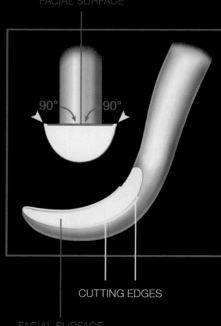

FACIAL SURFACE

90° 90°

CUTTING EDGES

FACIAL SURFACE

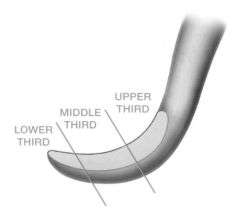

The working end can be divided into three parts:
• lower third
• middle third
• upper third

It is important to sharpen the entire cutting edge. It is possible to adjust sharpening pressure according to different degree of wear of the cutting edge.

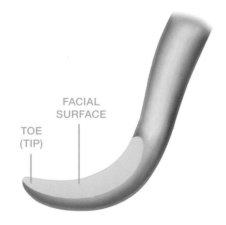

It is important to identify the parts of the working end:
• facial surface or frontal surface
• cutting edge or edges
• lateral surfaces
• back or bottom surface
• toe (tip)

The working end of the instrument can be rounded or pointed:

Both universal and area-specific curets always present a rounded toe (tip) and are semicircular in cross-section.

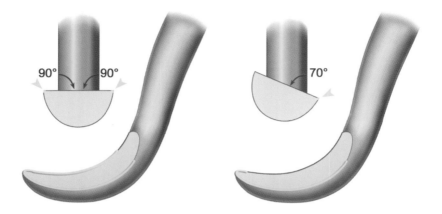

Sickle scalers have a pointed (tapered) tip, they have a so-called heel (the end of the blade on the shank side) and they are triangular in-cross-section.

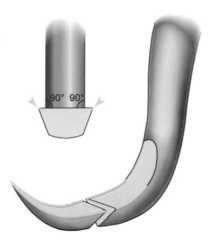

Universal and area-specific curets always have a rounded tip (toe).

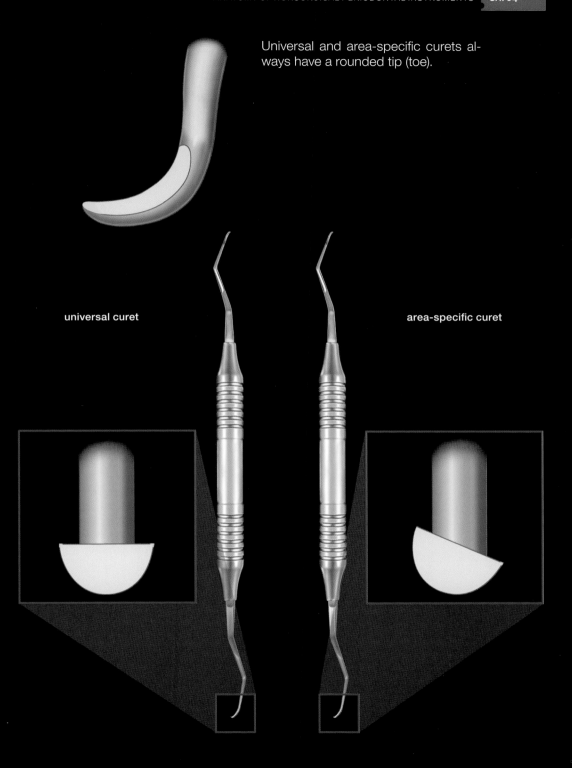

universal curet

area-specific curet

A sickle, whether straight or angulated, always presents a very tapered tip.

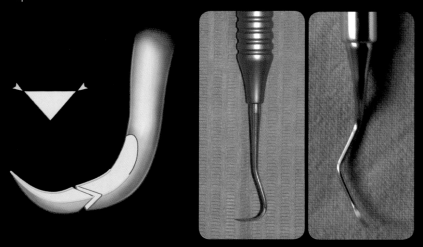

The working end of both Curets and Scalers can be:
• **Standard**
Not indicated for periodontal instrumentation of deep pocket, with vertical strokes.

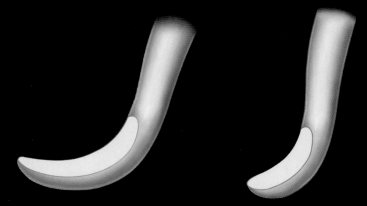

• **Mini**
Highly recommended for advanced periodontal instrumentation in deep narrow pockets but also indicated for routine maintenance therapy.
• **Micro-Mini**
Not as desirable as Mini instruments; In my opinion, the Micro Mini instruments tend to wear out very quickly because of their extremely reduced dimensions.

For calculus removal, the lower third of the working end is primarily used. A modified activation technique associated with vertical or oblique strokes is employed.[14]

In a correctly executed vertical stroke, the lower third of the working end of the instrument is adapted to the root surface and then the handle is moved away from the surface being instrumented, as illustrated in the following figures.

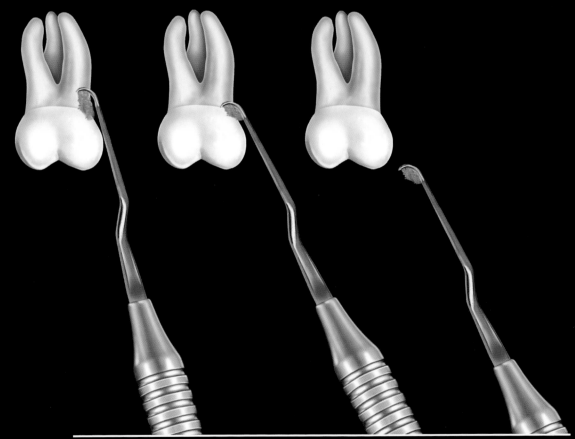

CORRECT

Conversely, all three thirds of the blade are used to perform a horizontal stroke. This stroke is usually the easiest for the operator to learn and is the stroke that determines an efficient nonsurgical periodontal instrumentation. The horizontal stroke allows removal of the entire calculus deposit with more predictable results because it reduces the risk of burnishing the calculus. Even in deep pockets strokes in a horizontal direction are very productive, compare to vertical and oblique strokes.

CORRECT

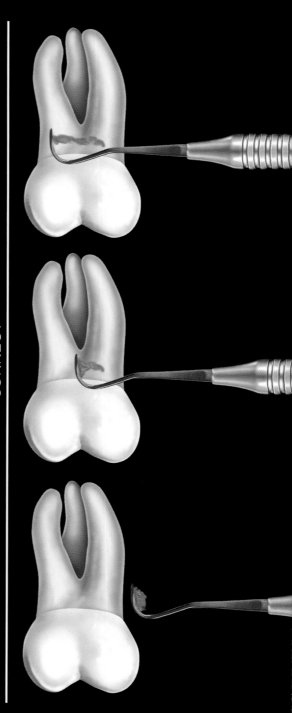

"Burnishing" Calculus is produced when the periodontal instrument slides over the deposits, merely smoothing and only partially removing them, leaving a residual layer of deposits on the root surface after the instrumentation. Burnished calculus can be the result of wrong working angulations, or of an incorrect technique in which the curet is simply drawn in a coronal direction rather than moved away from the instrumented surface as previously described.

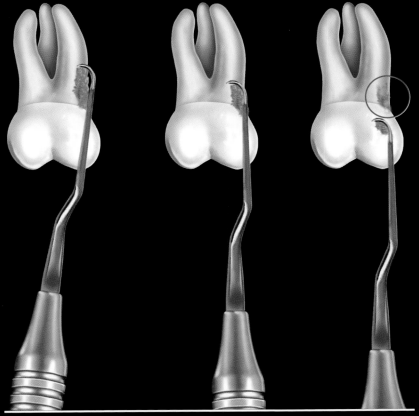

INCORRECT

It is possible to burnish a calcified deposit if one performs an incorrect nonsurgical periodontal instrumentation stroke or also if unsharpened instruments are used.

Residual deposits of burnished calculus jeopardize complete healing of an instrumented site. This concept confirms the importance of constant and frequent sharpening to support effective instrumentation.

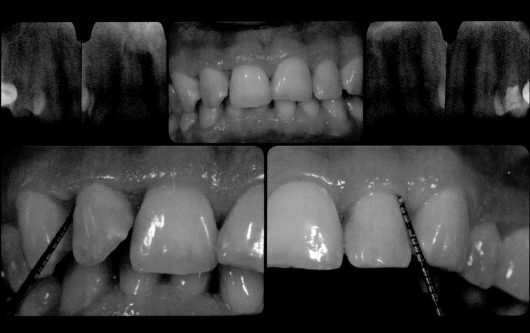

A patient presented several months after nonsurgical periodontal therapy was performed in another dental office. Radiographs taken at the initial patient visit show the presence of residual subgingival calculus on the interproximal surfaces of the anterior teeth. During professional nonsurgical periodontal instrumentation, the calcified deposits were completely removed in the maxillary left quadrant but only partially removed in the maxillary right quadrant. Posttreatment photographs show appropriate healing of tissues surrounding the anterior left dentition with well-represented papillae; in the maxillary right quadrant, healing is less satisfactory and, as a result, the papillae are not as much defined. Residual calculus has resulted in persistent inflammation.

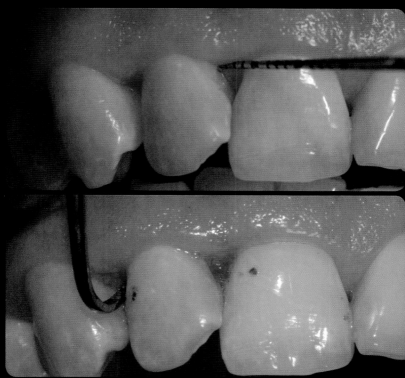

Using well-sharpened instruments, residual, burnished calculus deposits were removed during follow-up nonsurgical periodontal therapy.

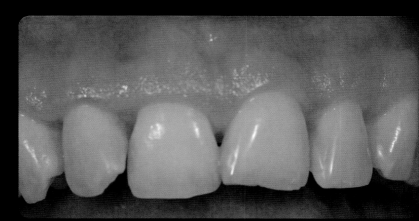

At the next follow-up appointment, improvement in the esthetics of the patient's smile is noted, with better-defined papillae in both quadrants. The healing process was favored by a more complete and accurate instrumentation and by the use of well-sharpened instruments.

STANDARD AND RIGID INSTRUMENTS

Another essential characteristic of all periodontal instruments: the tip of the instrument must fall on the vertical axis of the handle.

It is essential to check whether this feature is observed, when purchasing new instruments, especially those which are attractively priced or those from an unknown or substandard brand.

When ordering new instruments, it is recommended to require specifically rigid ones. The instruments can be: standard, rigid and in some cases even extra-rigid. What differs is mainly the flexibility of the shank, the instrument has a standard shank somewhat flexible, in case of particularly stubborn deposits, it tends to bend, mal opposing the pressure required to remove the tartar. A standard instrument is indicated for follow-up instrumentation and for the removal of light-to-moderate deposits. Conversely in case of advanced periodontal instrumentation, it is advantageous to prefer rigid instruments that can better transfer the pressure, exerted by the arm, through the shank to the cutting edge. Rigid instruments can be used with great profit even in the case of very small deposits.

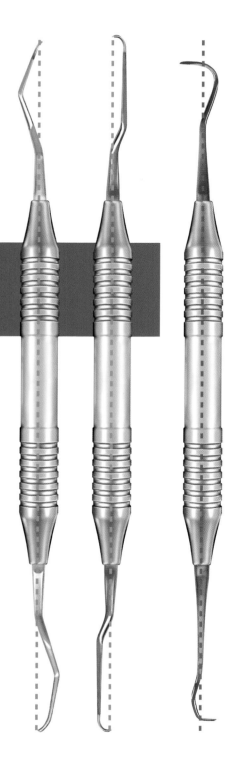

CLASSIFICATION OF NONSURGICAL PERIODONTAL INSTRUMENTS

Periodontal non surgical instruments can be categorized in:

SICKLE SCALER

1. it is always a universal instrument,
2. it presents two cutting edges on each working end for a total of four cutting edges,
3. in cross-section, the triangular tip becomes rounded towards the back,
4. it can be used in any tooth surface,
5. its pronounced, tapered tip must not be sharpened (unlike the toe of a curet) if its characteristic shape, created by sharpening the two cutting edges of the working end, is to be maintained,
6. it can have a straight or angulated shank.

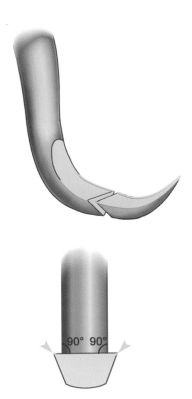

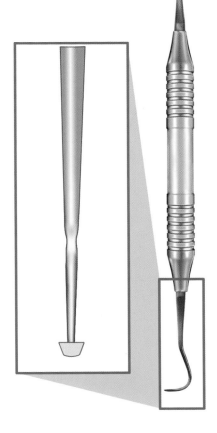

Scaler with an angulated shank

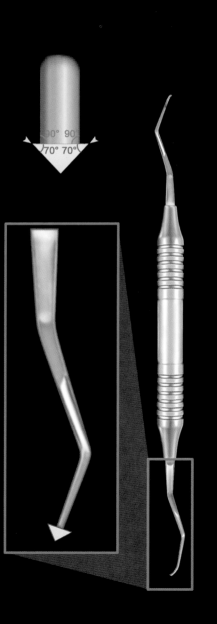

Scaler with a straight shank

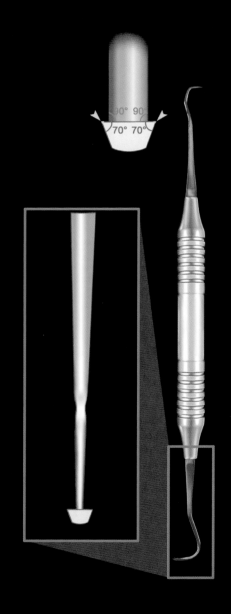

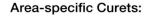

CURETS

Universal Curets:

1. have two cutting edges on each working end opposite the handle for a total of four cutting edges.

2. can be used on any tooth surface.

3. the face (frontal surface) is at a 90-degree angle to the lower shank, which creates two cutting edges.

4. have an angulated shank, with the exception of the straight-shanked 5/6 Langer curet (the use of the 5/6 Langer curet is not recommended by the author).

Area-specific Curets:

1. one cutting edge on each working end opposite the handle for a total of two cutting edges.

2. can only be used on specific surfaces; for example, the 11/12 curet is used to instrument the mesial surface of posterior teeth.

3. Gracey Curet blades are honed so that the face is "off-set" at approximately 70-degree to the lower part of the shank, outlining a higher edge and a lower edge.

4. the lower edge is always the cutting edge.

5. another method to determine which of the two is the correct cutting edge to adapt to the tooth: the blade should be held face up and parallel with the floor, the larger outer curve of the working end is always the correct cutting edge.

6. can have a straight or angulated shank.

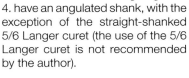

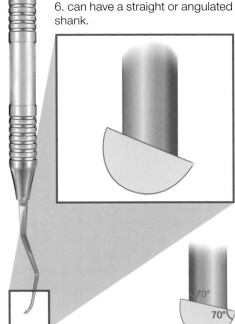

FILES

Hirschfeld periodontal files

The file is an instrument with multiple cutting edges.[7] The Hirschfeld periodontal files are classified as 3/7, 5/11, and 9/10. These miniaturized files are indicated as finishing instruments, for example to smooth down a root surface, which appears somewhat irregularly rough, even after intensive instrumentation. But they are also used in initial nonsurgical periodontal instrumentation of narrow deep pockets, where removal of calculus is accomplished by crushing or fragmentation.[15] Push and pull strokes should be used to activate these instruments.[7] A dedicated instrument called file sharpener must be purchased and used to sharpen these periodontal files (see Chapter 3, "Sharpening Materials").

Roncati files

The Roncati file is a newly designed nonsurgical periodontal instrument that is used for the same indications as the Hirschfeld files. The Roncati file has an advantage over the Hirschfeld file in that it does not need to be sharpened because it has a diamond-coated working surface.

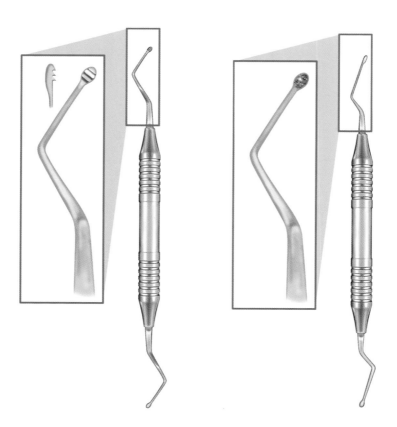

HOES

These instruments are included in this text for completeness sake; however, they are not used routinely by the author. Therefore, their sharpening or use will not be illustrated. Ultrasonic instruments or other nonsurgical periodontal instruments discussed in this text are preferred over hoes.

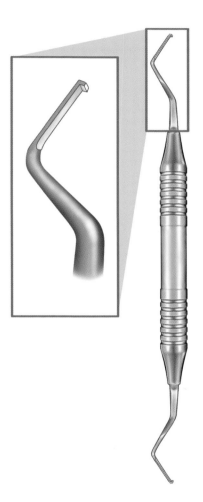

For routine nonsurgical periodontal instrumentation, **universal** and **area-specific instruments** are most frequently used.

UNIVERSAL INSTRUMENTS	AREA-SPECIFIC INSTRUMENTS
Universal curets and sickle scalers	Area-specific curets

UNIVERSAL INSTRUMENTS

1 • SICKLE SCALERS
   Available with a straight or an angulated lower shank.

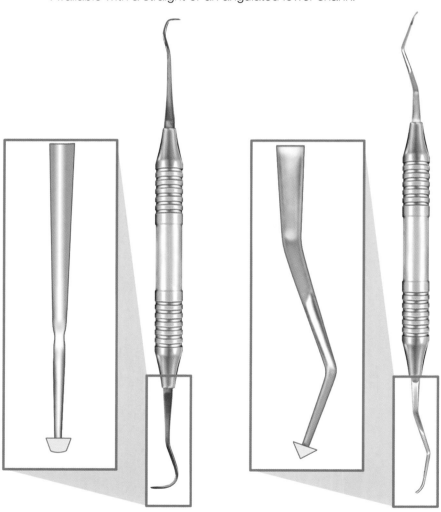

2 • UNIVERSAL CURETS

Available with a straight or an angulated lower shank.

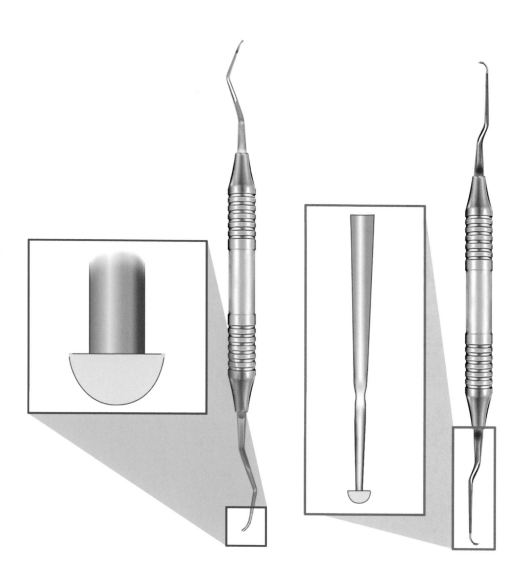

The only universal curet with a straight lower shank is the Langer curet 5/6. This curet was designed by Dr Burton Langer for anterior tooth surfaces instrumentation. Because the Langer curet has two cutting edges, use of this instrument with vertical strokes on anterior tooth surfaces in not recommended.

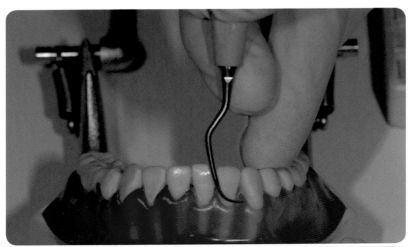

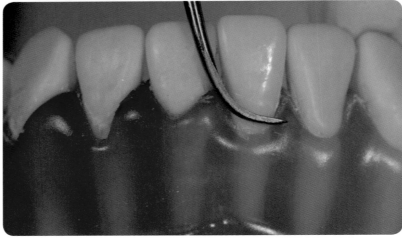

In particular, the 5/6 Langer curet is disproportionately greater than the mesiodistal dimensions of the anterior teeth, so vertical strokes with this instrument will increase the chances of tissue trauma.
If the 5/6 Langer curet is to be used clinically, it is recommended to limit its use to horizontal strokes only.
Anyhow I do not like the Langer 5/6 curet.

ALL UNIVERSAL INSTRUMENTS ARE SHARPENED WITH THE STONE AT A 20-DEGREE ANGLE TO THE LOWER SHANK.

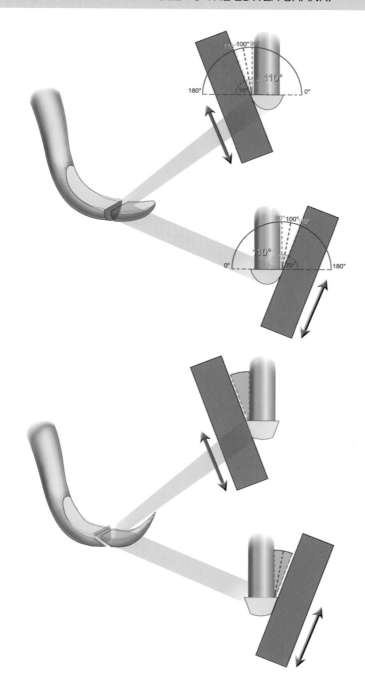

AREA-SPECIFIC INSTRUMENTS

1 • GRACEY CURETS
The 1/2, 3/4, 5/6 7/8, and 9/10 Gracey curets all have a straight lower shank.

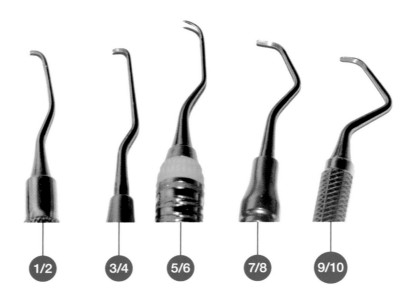

1/2   3/4   5/6   7/8   9/10

In my opinion, the 1/2 curet is primarily indicated for the instrumentation. The 3/4 and 5/6 curets can also be used with vertical strokes, especially in their Mini versions. The 7/8 and, particularly, the 9/10 curets have very broad shanks, and therefore their use should be limited to horizontal strokes mainly on posterior teeth.

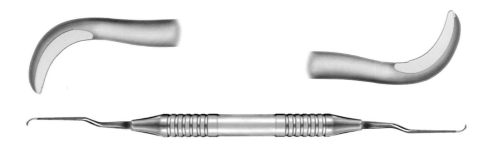

The 11/12 and 15/16 Gracey curets have an angulated lower shank. Both are used on the mesial surfaces of posterior teeth.

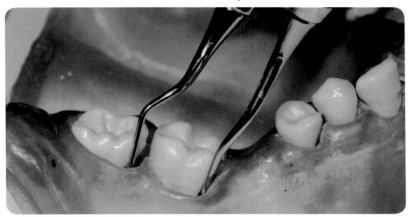

The 15/16 curet has a more highly angulated shank than the 11/12, favoring its insertion in more posterior areas, according to the manufacturers; however, the 11/12 curet is more commonly used. Extraoral fulcrums, non dominant hand fulcrum reinforcement or alternative finger rests can aid instrumentation in the most posterior areas, making the use of the Gracey curet 11/12 very effective in advanced non surgical periodontal instrumentation.

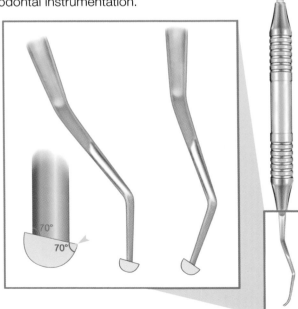

The 13/14 and 17/18 curets also have an angulated lower shank; they are both used to instrument the distal surfaces of the posterior teeth.

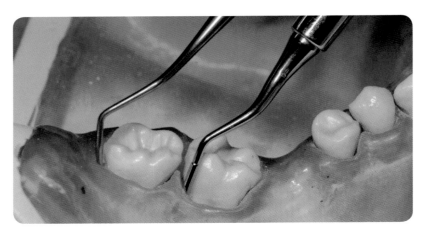

The 13/14 curet, when used with an extraoral fulcrum, can efficiently reach any distal surface and is preferred over the 17/18 curet.

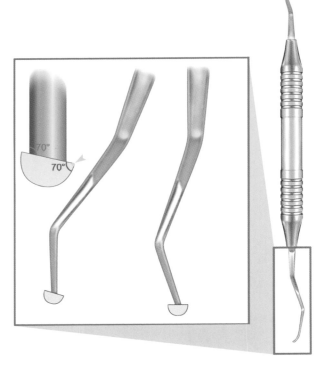

2 • CURVETTES

Curvettes are area-specific curets available in four versions: sub-zero, 1/2, 11/12, and 13/14. Their working ends have reduced dimensions and are somewhat curvilinear. The lower part of the shank is notched at 5 mm and at 10 mm. Moreover, the shank is aligned more closely with the handle than on the Gracey curet.

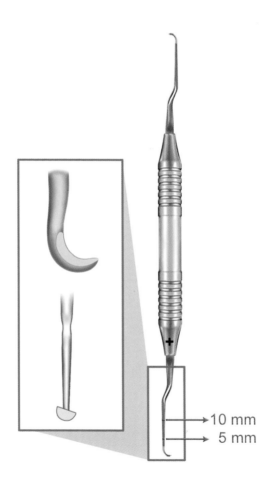

→ 10 mm
→ 5 mm

THE MINIMAL NONSURGICAL PERIODONTAL INSTRUMENT KIT

Nonsurgical periodontal instrumentation can be proficiently performed with a minimum number of instruments. In addition to a dental mirror, a periodontal probe, gauzes, and a sharpening stone, the tray might hold three other instruments:

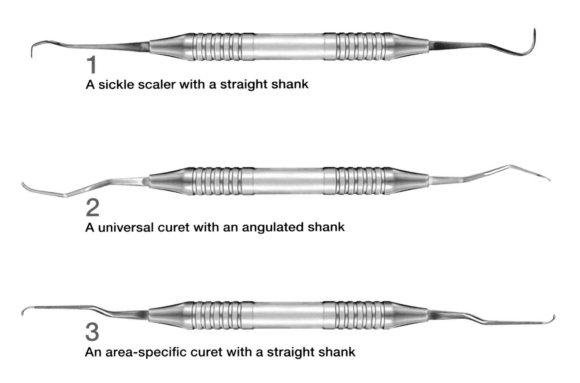

1

A sickle scaler with a straight shank

2

A universal curet with an angulated shank

3

An area-specific curet with a straight shank

A few well-sharpened instruments and a careful technique are sufficient for effective nonsurgical periodontal instrumentation. The objective is to efficiently remove all calcified deposits without burnishing them and to respect tissue integrity as well as patient's comfort.

SHARPENING ERRORS

05

GET SHARP
NONSURGICAL PERIODONTAL INSTRUMENT SHARPENING

DO NOT SHARPEN EVERY INSTRUMENT USING THE SAME ANGLE BETWEEN STONE AND HANDLE

The three instruments of the minimal kit[14] will be examined as representative of the most frequently used instruments.

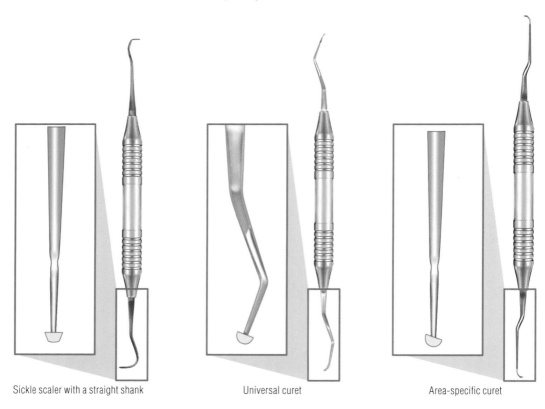

Sickle scaler with a straight shank   Universal curet   Area-specific curet

Each of these instruments has different characteristics. The most frequent **error** is positioning the stone at the same angle, usually 45 degrees, in relation to the handle of every instrument. While it is true that all nonsurgical periodontal instruments must be sharpened at **a fixed angle**, this angle is **not** formed by the handle and the stone and, above all, is **not** a 45-degree angle.

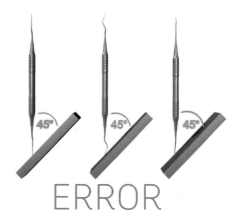

ERROR

If the three instruments are examined in cross-section, the cutting edge/s, marked with a red triangle, is/are always between the facial and lateral surfaces of the working end.

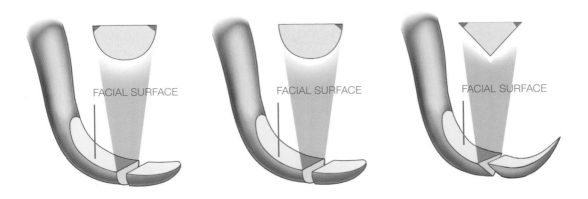

The universal curet and the sickle scaler have two cutting edges, while the area-specific curet has only one blade. In all three instruments, internal angles of 70 degrees are formed where the facial surface meet the lateral surface at the cutting edge.

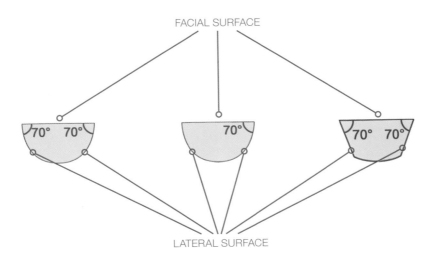

To sharpen the cutting edge, the lateral surface must be reduced by positioning the stone at the correct angle so the instrument dimensions are reduced with no proportions modification.

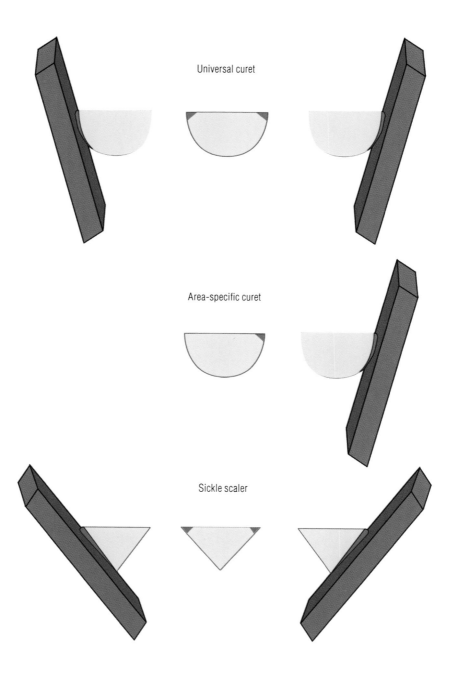

Universal curet

Area-specific curet

Sickle scaler

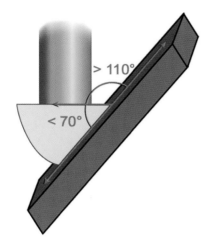

INCORRECT

If the stone is positioned at greater than 110 degrees in relation to the face of the working end, the resulting angle of the cutting edge will be less than 70 degrees. Initially, the instrument will appear to be well sharpened, but the cutting edge will tend to lose its sharpness rapidly. Moreover, the instrument will become thinner and more fragile.

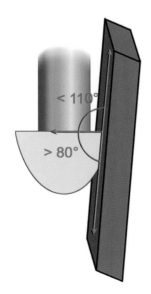

INCORRECT

If the stone is positioned at less than 110 degrees in relation to the face of the working end, the resulting angle of the cutting edge will be greater than 70 degrees, and the original form of the instrument will again be altered. A sharpened cutting edge will be obtained, but its bulkiness will cause difficulty during instrumentation. Heavy lateral pressure is required to remove deposits and calculus removal is often incomplete.[7]

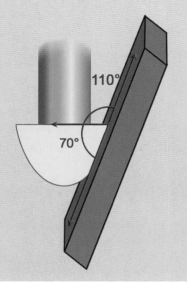

CORRECT

If the stone is positioned at precisely 110 degrees in relation to the facial surface of the working end, the lateral surface is properly and consistently reduced.

Therefore, the stone must be **always** positioned at 110 degrees **in relation to the facial surface**[1,7,12,15] when sharpening all nonsurgical periodontal instruments.

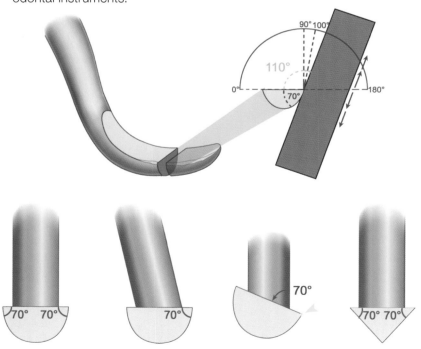

The facial surface may be at a **right angle** or **offset** (beveled at 70° angle to the lower part of the shank).

It is fundamental to focus closely on the lower part of the shank.[14]

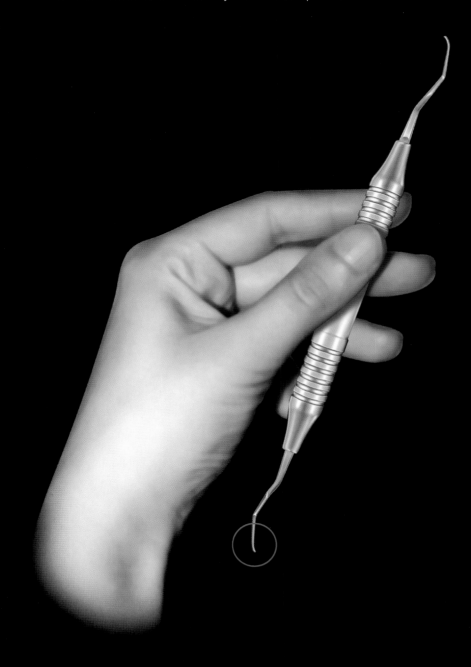

The **shank** can be straight or angulated.

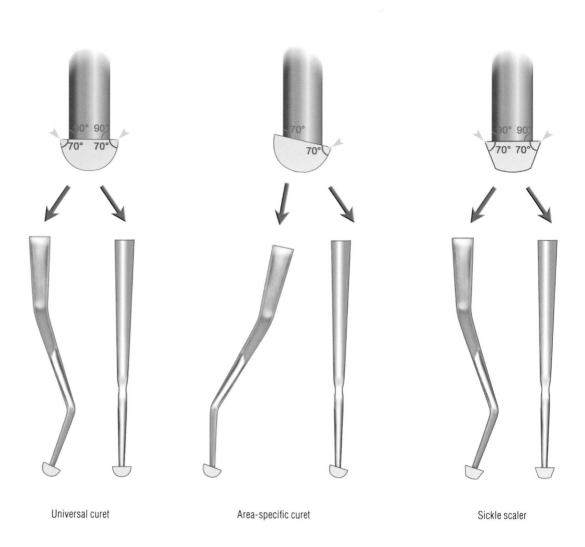

Universal curet   Area-specific curet   Sickle scaler

Therefore, to maintain an angle of 110 degrees between the facial surface and the stone, the position of the handle will change in relation to the stone, depending on the instrument.

Note how the position of the handle varies between a **universal curet** with a straight shank and one with an angulated shank, although the angle of 20 degrees between the lower shank and the stone does not change.

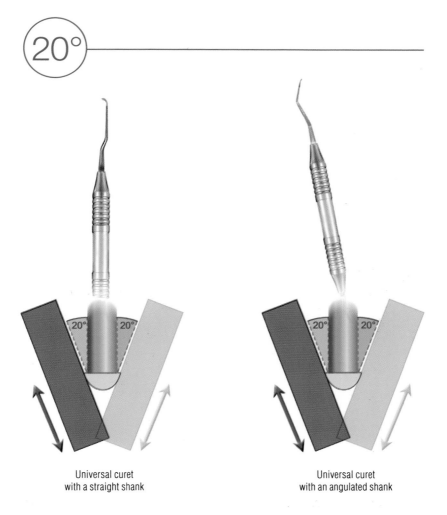

Universal curet
with a straight shank

Universal curet
with an angulated shank

Similarly, the position of the handle varies when sharpening a **scaler** with a straight shank and a scaler with an angulated shank.

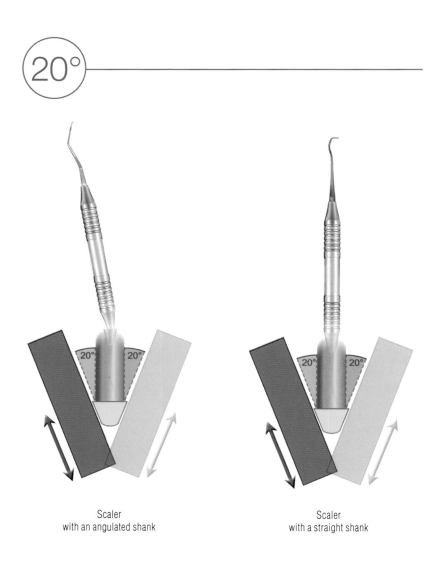

Scaler
with an angulated shank

Scaler
with a straight shank

The angle between the stone and the lower shank is always 20 degrees because the scaler is always a universal instrument.

For the **area-specific curets**, the angle between the stone and the lower shank is always 40 degrees. Whereas the position of the handle in relation to the stone varies for different Gracey Curets.

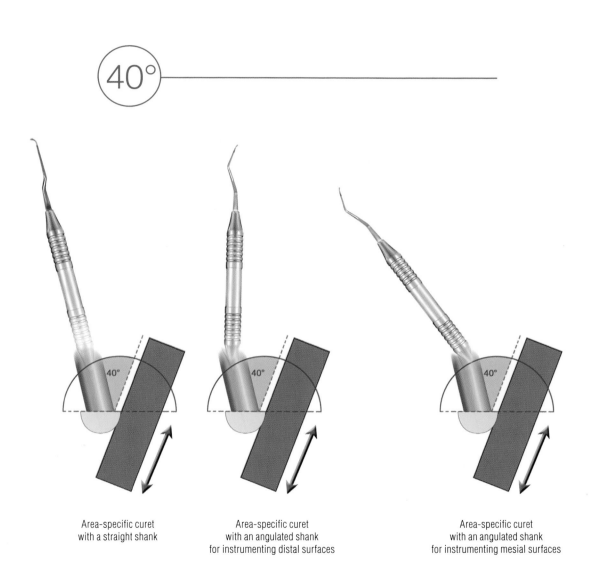

40°

Area-specific curet
with a straight shank

Area-specific curet
with an angulated shank
for instrumenting distal surfaces

Area-specific curet
with an angulated shank
for instrumenting mesial surfaces

DO NOT FORGET SHARPENING THE TIP OF THE CURET, WHETHER UNIVERSAL OR AREA-SPECIFIC

All **curets**, whether universal or area-specific, terminate in a rounded toe (Tip).

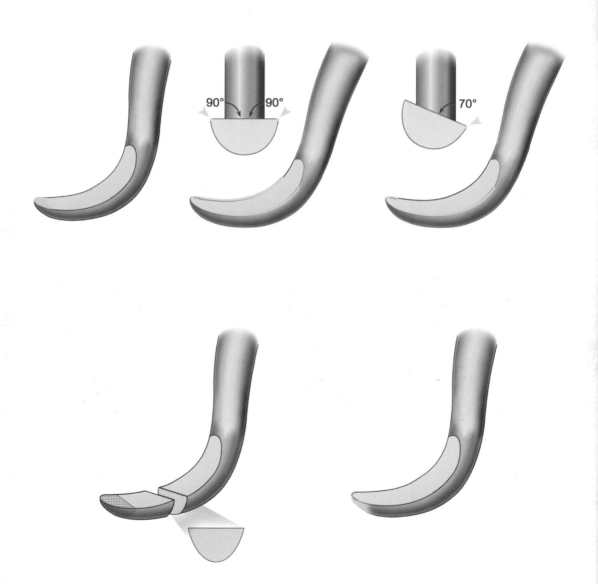

In the moving flat stone/stationary instrument sharpening technique, the whole cutting edge of the instrument is progressively sharpened by incremental movements of the stone, so that sharpening continues around the curved toe. Follow the cutting edge from heel to toe, applying several strokes to each millimeters.[1] The original contours are preserved, and the toe remains well-rounded with this technique. Decrease the facial surface/stone angle to 45° at the toe.[7]

CORRECT

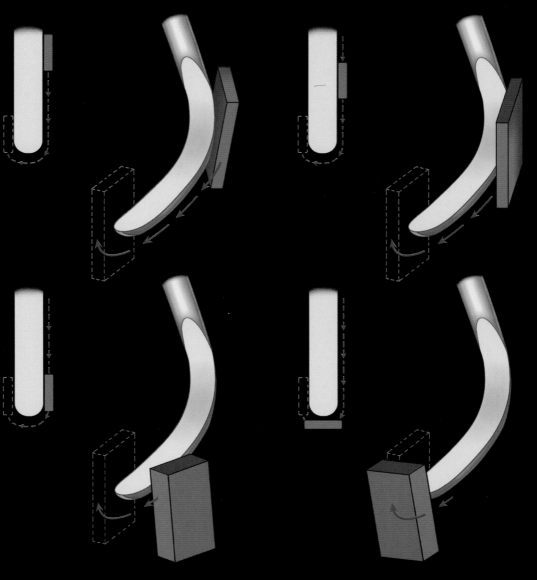

Conversely, if the operator stops incremental sharpening too soon before approaching the toe (tip), the instrument will become deformed and will take on the pointed profile of a sickle scaler rather than preserving the original round design typical of a curet. This type of missharpening can also be detected by viewing the instrument from directly above the face of the blade.[7]

INCORRECT

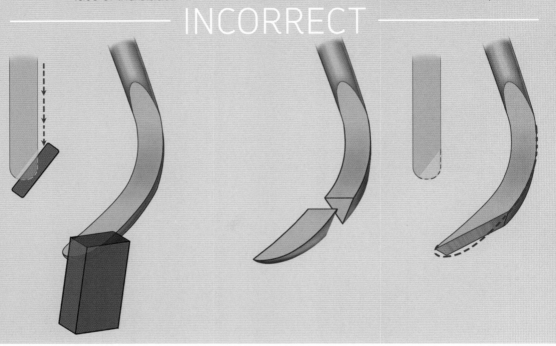

The dimensions of a well-sharpened instrument will be progressively reduced, while the proportions of the original instrument will be maintained.

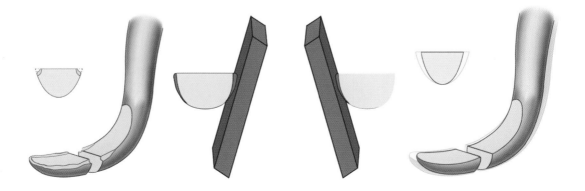

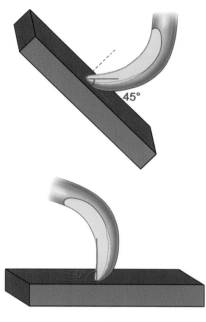

To avoid this frequent mistake, the toe (tip), of the instrument should be recontoured and rounded before sharpening the rest of the cutting edge.

The toe (tip), of all curets is beveled at an angle of 45 degrees; the stone must be held at this angle when sharpening around the toe.

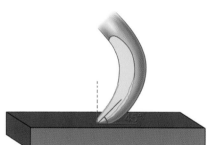

If we adapt the stationary flat stone, moving instrument technique, the instrument will initially be positioned with the handle parallel to the stone and with the toe (tip) placed at 90 degrees to the stone surface.

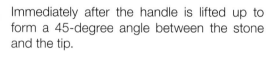

Immediately after the handle is lifted up to form a 45-degree angle between the stone and the tip.

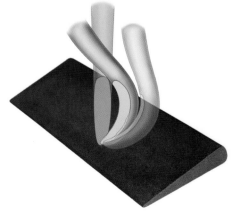

Short, continuous sharpening movements are made while maintaining a constant 45-degree angle, until the toe (tip) has been satisfactorily reshaped. At this point, the toe may appear somewhat squared, so several short lateral strokes may be necessary to restore the terminal curvature of the toe, while progressively and gradually rolling the instrument between finger pads.

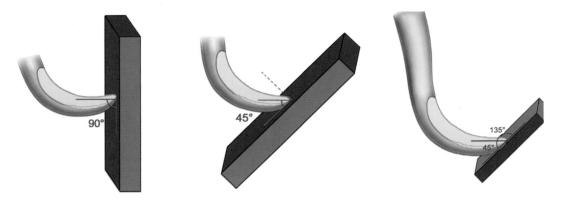

In case the moving flat stone, stationary instrument technique is implemented the stone is held with the dominant hand, it will initially be positioned at a right angle to the toe with the handle of the instrument parallel to the stone. The stone is then inclined 45 degrees before starting sharpening movements to recontour the toe (tip).

The operator begins sharpening with short, well controlled and continuous up and down strokes, while paying particular attention to maintaining the 45-degree angle between the **stone and the tip**. The tip might result somewhat squared, so it must be rounded to maintain the proper terminal curvature and this can be accomplished by revolving the stone while sharpen with slow, gradual, and progressive lateral strokes around the tip.

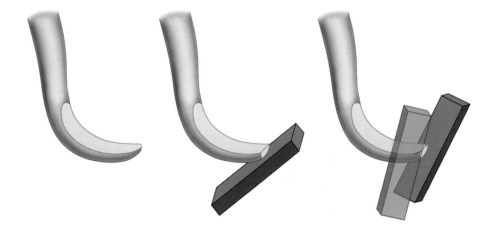

DO NOT SHARPEN THE INSTRUMENT FRONTAL SURFACE

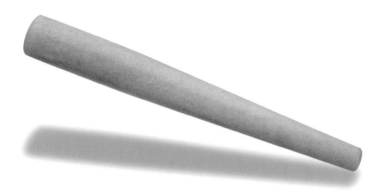

Sharpening cone: a cylindrical Arkansan or India stone is applied to a face of a curet. The stone is positioned to fit the curvature of the surface to be.[1] Rotate stone counterclockwise over the instrument with even firm pressure.[1]

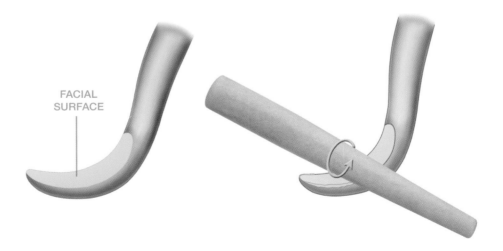

FACIAL
SURFACE

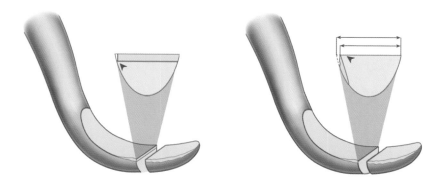

The cylindrical stone grinds metal from the facial surface to restore the cutting edge of the instrument. This technique is not recommended because it produces is a thinner, more fragile instrument, increasing the risk of fracture during calculus removal.[13,16] Therefore cautiousness is highly suggested in case of utilization.

The cylindrical stone is indicated for the removal of "wire edge": small, thin filaments of metal projecting from the cutting edge[6] that may develop during the sharpening process.

However, use of the cylindrical stone is optional.

CORRECT SHARPENING TECHNIQUES

06

GET SHARP
NONSURGICAL PERIODONTAL INSTRUMENT SHARPENING

The 110-degree **sharpening angle is the only correct one**. The angle between the stone and the face of the blade should always be maintained at 110 degrees, regardless of the sharpening technique implemented, for the following nonsurgical periodontal instruments: **curets**, both universal and area-specific, and **scalers**, both angulated or straight.

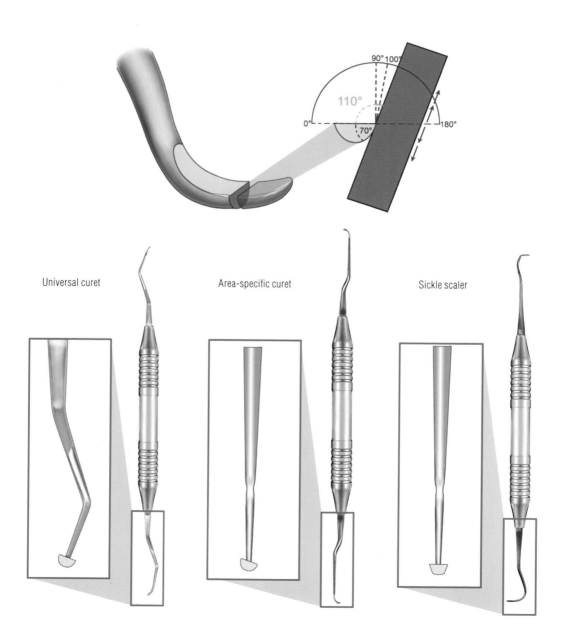

Universal curet

Area-specific curet

Sickle scaler

To avoid mistakes, it is essential to be mindful of the following: The 110-degree **sharpening angle** is formed by the **stone** and the **facial surface** of the instrument cutting edge. Because this angle is difficult to visualize, recurrently the clinician might wrongly focus on the more evident angle between the instrument handle and the stone. Lack of awareness of this significant concept leads to frequent sharpening errors.

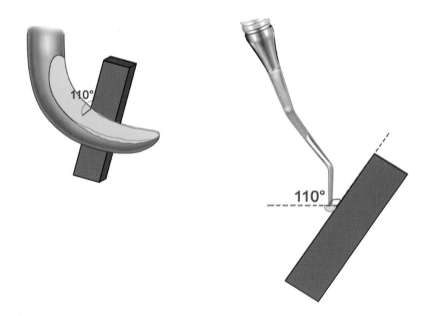

The correct 110-degree angle is always formed by the stone and the facial surface, both for **curets** and **scalers**.

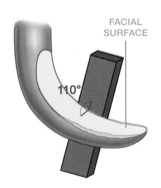

Universal curet

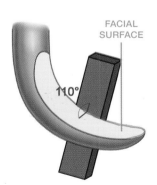

Area-specific curet

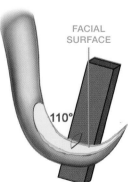

Sickle scaler

SHARPENING METHODS

There are two techniques for manual sharpening of instruments: the *stationary stone/moving instrument sharpening method and the stationary instrument/moving stone technique.* Both are adequate for obtaining a satisfactory degree of sharpening for all nonsurgical periodontal instruments.

The choice of the more suitable technique rests with the operator, depending on his or her manual skills and preference.

Before choosing one technique over the other, it is recommended to practice both.

It is essential to remember that the sharpening angle is always 110 degrees. The detailed instructions that follow will show how this principle is put into practice for each class of nonsurgical periodontal instruments (**curets** and **scalers**), using both techniques.

STATIONARY STONE/MOVING INSTRUMENT TECHNIQUE

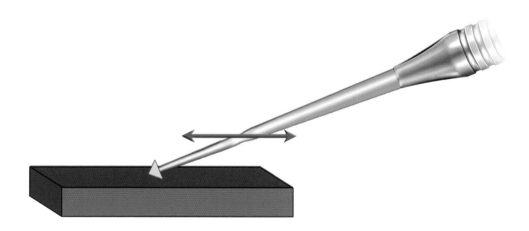

Prepare the stone and place it flat on a steady working surface. The movement of the instrument is shown by the blue arrow.

40° Area-specific curet

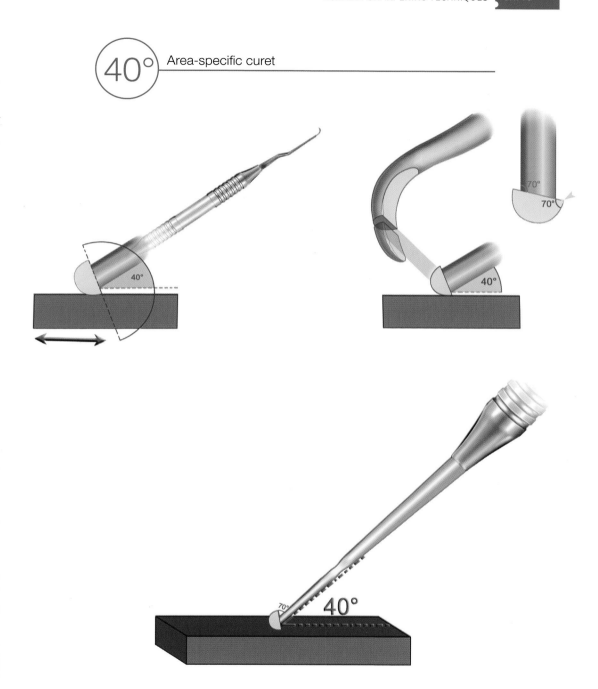

20°   Universal curet

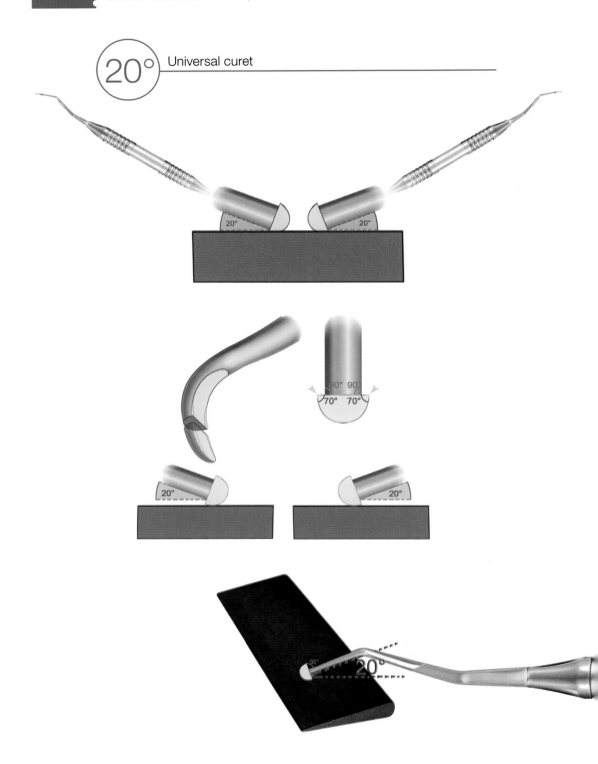

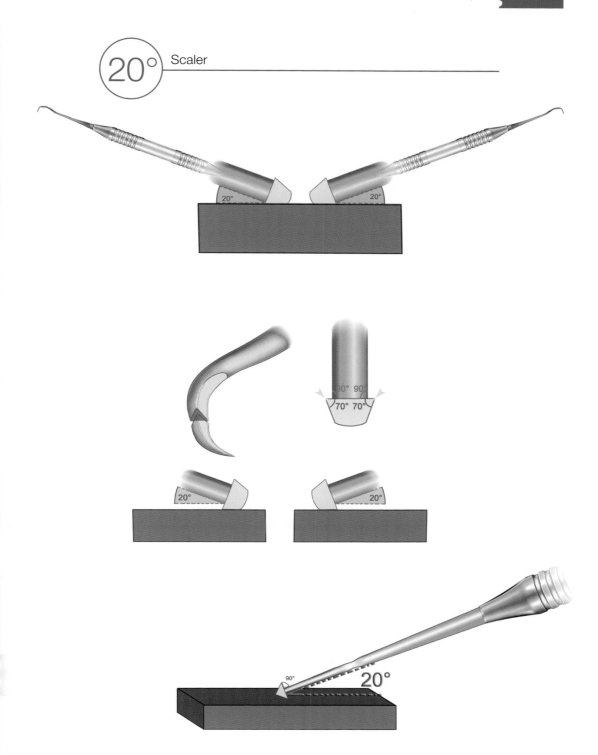

20° Scaler

STATIONARY INSTRUMENT/MOVING STONE TECHNIQUE

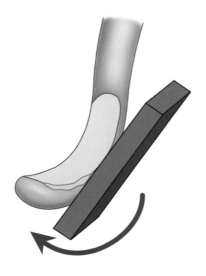

In the stationary instrument/moving stone sharpening method, the instrument is firmly grasped in the operator's nondominant hand while the stone is moved by the dominant hand (blue arrow).

 40° Area-specific curet

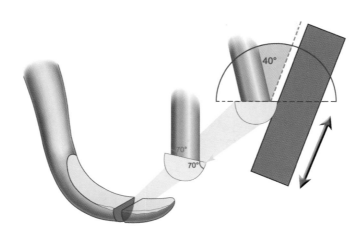

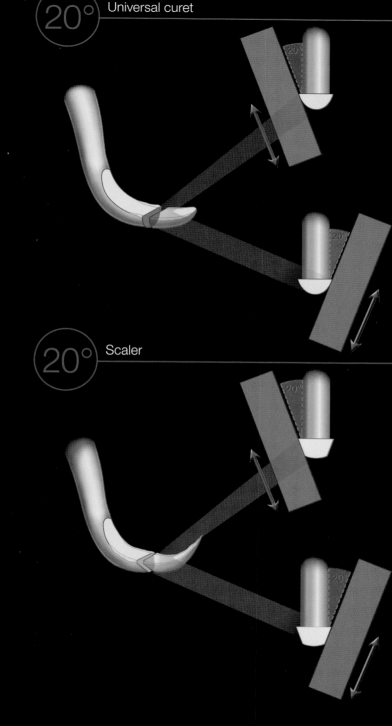

Universal curet

20°

Scaler

20°

SHARPENING THE UNIVERSAL CURET

Stationary instrument/moving stone technique

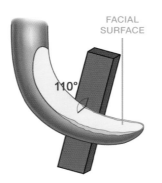

The correct angle between the stone and the facial surface is always 110 degrees. Practically, though, it is necessary to create a **20-degree angle between the stone and the lower shank** of the instrument to obtain a 110-degree angle between the stone and the facial surface.

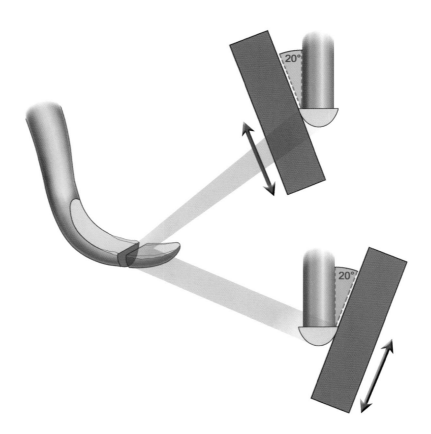

As fully illustrated on Chapter 4, the angle between the facial surface and the lower shank of all universal curets is, by definition, 90 degrees, consequently, to maintain the correct 110-degree angle between the instrument face and the stone, it is simply necessary to create a 20 degree angle between the lower shank and the stone. The illustration below shows the 20-degree angle between the stone and the lower shank, which is much easier to picture than the 110-degree angle between the facial surface and the stone.

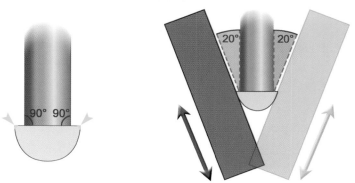

Both cutting edges at each end of the handle have to be sharpened. It is important to remember that the universal curet can have a straight shank, such as the 5/6 Langer curet, or an angulated shank. As a result, the position of the handle will vary among instruments, in order to maintain the same 20 degrees angle between the stone and the instrument lower shank, as illustrated in the figure.

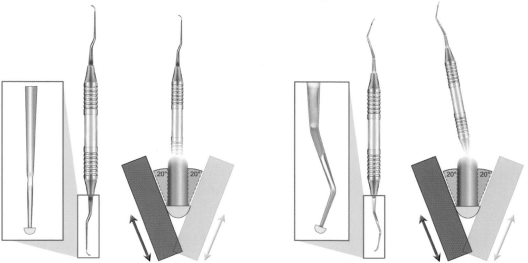

5/6 Langer curet   Curet with an angulated shank

Stationary stone/moving instrument technique

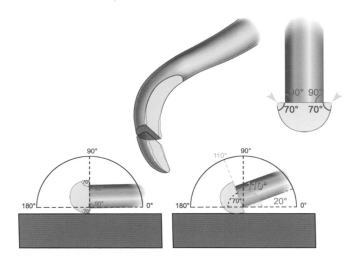

In this technique, the 110-degree angle between the stone and the facial surface of the instrument must also be observed. Hold the stone flat against on a horizontal working surface with one hand while with the opposite hand the instrument is moved across it.

To maintain the 110-degree angle between the stone and the facial surface, a 20-degree angle is established between the stone and the lower part of the shank, as shown in the figure below.

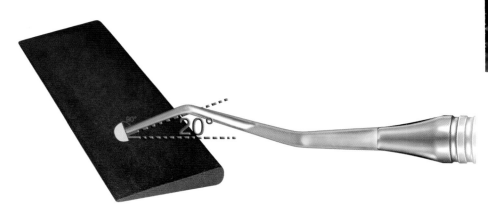

The stone is positioned on a stable working surface and a 20-degree angle between the stone and the lower shank is created. To facilitate the procedure, a useful suggestion is to place the stone overhanging on the edge of the working surface while the lower part of the shank is initially laid down on the short side of the stone and immediately after slightly lifted, as shown in the figure, to maintain the correct 20-degrees angle between the stone and the instrument lower shank.

Both cutting edges on either end of curet handle are sharpened while observing the 20-degree angle between the lower part of the shank and the stone.

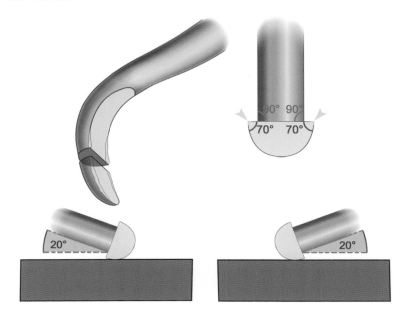

If a **universal curet** with an angulated shank is sharpened using the stationary instrument/moving stone technique, difficulties may be greater.

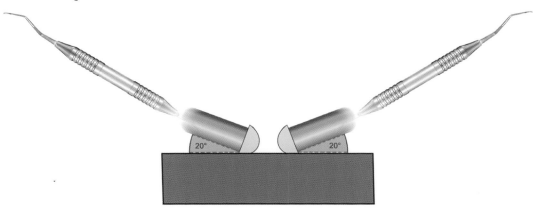

Therefore, the stationary stone/moving instrument technique is recommended for sharpening universal instruments.

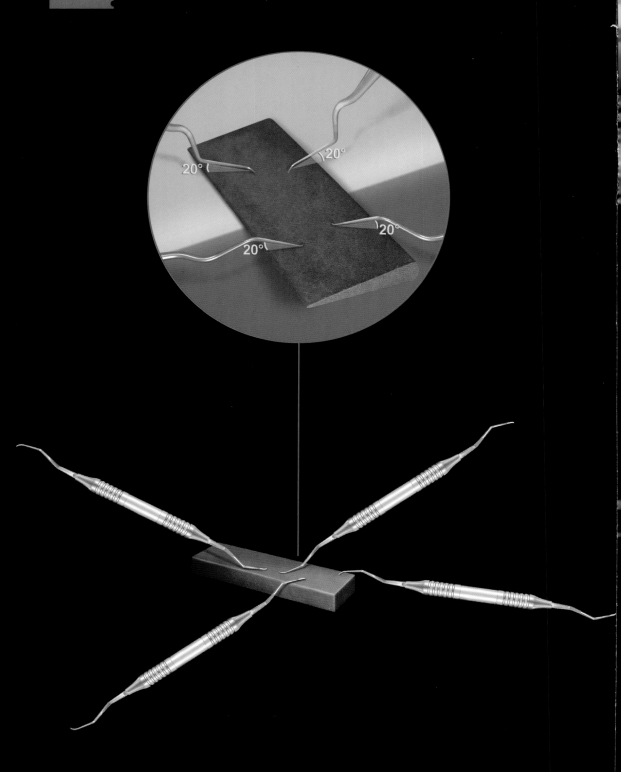

SHARPENING THE AREA-SPECIFIC CURET

Stationary instrument/moving stone technique

Like the universal instruments, for the **area-specific curet** the correct sharpening angle between the stone and the facial surface is 110 degrees. It is important to remember that only one cutting edge is sharpened on either end of the handle.

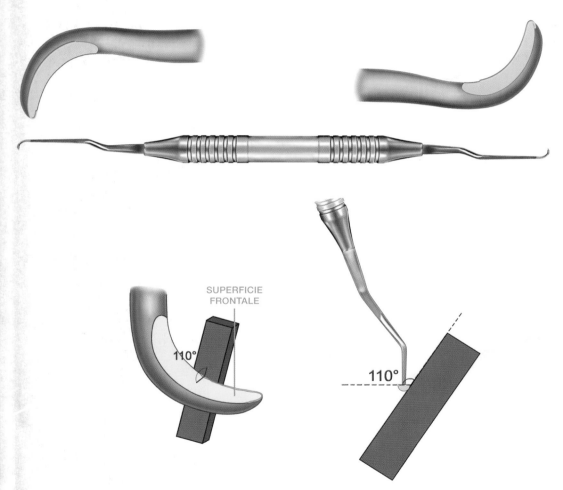

SUPERFICIE FRONTALE

110°

110°

Right in order to maintain the 110-degree correct angle between the stone and the facial surface, a 40-degree angle is established between the stone and the lower shank.

There is only one cutting edge to sharpen on each end of the handle. The figure shows the 40-degree angle between the lower shank and the stone.

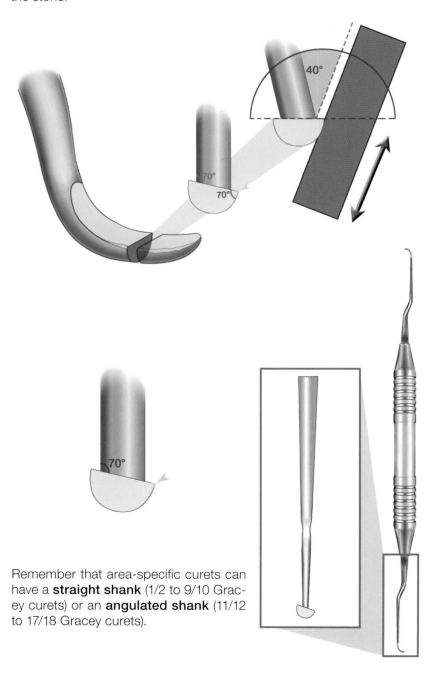

Remember that area-specific curets can have a **straight shank** (1/2 to 9/10 Gracey curets) or an **angulated shank** (11/12 to 17/18 Gracey curets).

Area-specific curet
for mesial surfaces

Area-specific curet
for distal surfaces

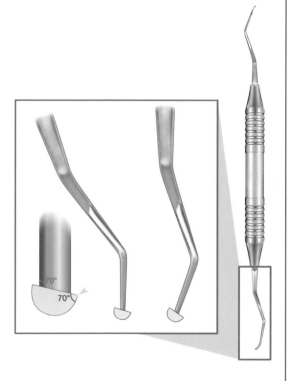

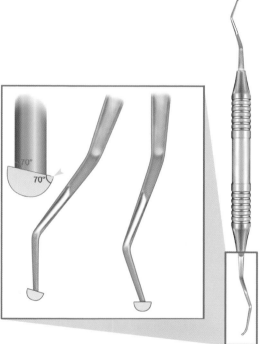

As a result, please note how the position of the handle will significantly vary among instruments so as to maintain the 40-degree angle between the stone and the lower part of instrument shank, as well as the correct 110-degree angle between the face of the blade and the stone, as illustrated in the figure.

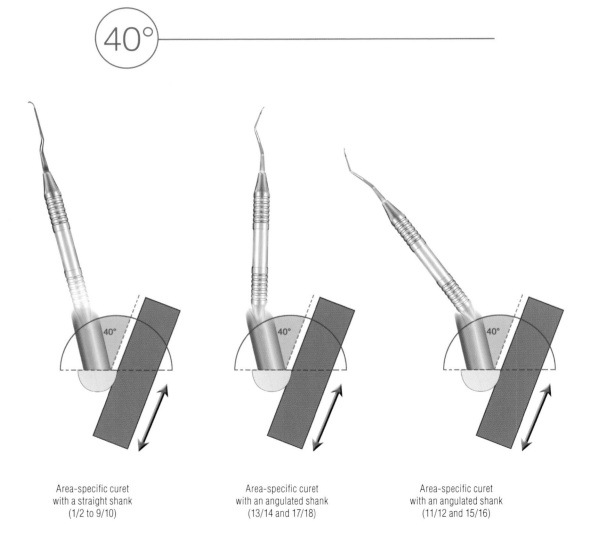

40°

| Area-specific curet with a straight shank (1/2 to 9/10) | Area-specific curet with an angulated shank (13/14 and 17/18) | Area-specific curet with an angulated shank (11/12 and 15/16) |

Stationary stone /moving instrument technique

The 40-degree angle between the lower shank and the stone is also maintained in this sharpening technique.

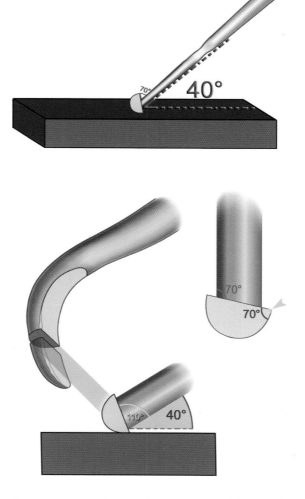

After stabilizing the stone on a horizontal steady working surface, a 40-degree angle is created between the lower shank and the stone. This preserves the correct 110-degree angle between the facial surface and the stone, as shown in the figure.

It is important to note that, when sharpening with the stationary stone/moving instrument technique, the position of the handle varies greatly in relation to the stone while maintaining the 40-degree angle between the lower shank and the stone. For all **area-specific curets**, only one cutting edge is sharpened on each end of the handle. Note how in the picture the yellow arch represent the 110-degree angle, which embraces the 40-degree angle + the 70-degree angle (between the lower shank and the face of the blade, as shown in the figures at pg.106).

Please note how the position of the handle will significantly vary among instruments so as to maintain the 40-degree angle between the stone and the lower part of instrument shank, as well as the correct 110-degree angle between the face of the blade and the stone, as illustrated in the figures. All Gracey Curets present only one cutting edge on each end of the handle, that has to be sharpen.

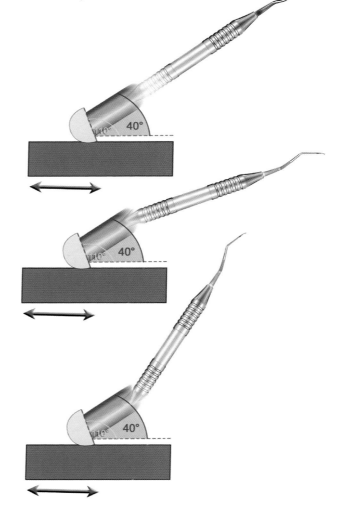

Area-specific curett
with a straight shank
(1/2 to 9/10)

Area-specific curett
with an angulated shank
(13/14 and 17/18)

Area-specific curett
with an angulated shank
(11/12 and 15/16)

SHARPENING THE SCALER

Stationary instrument/moving stone technique

The correct sharpening angle between the stone and the facial surface for sickle scalers is as always 110 degrees. As fully illustrated on Chapter 4, the angle between the facial surface and the lower shank of all universal instruments (the sickle is always an universal instrument) is, by definition, 90 degrees, consequently, to maintain the correct 110-degree angle between the instrument face and the stone, it is simply necessary to create a 20 degree angle between the lower shank and the stone.

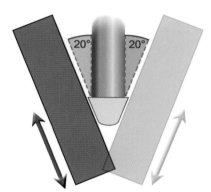

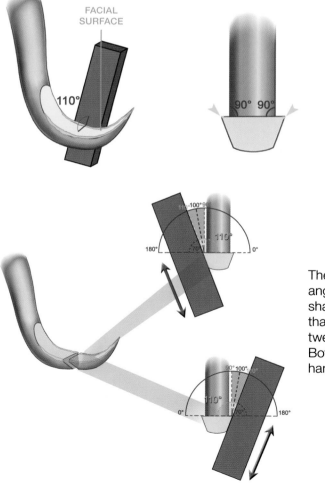

The illustration shows the 20-degree angle between the stone and the lower shank, which is much easier to picture than the correct 110-degree angle between the facial surface and the stone. Both cutting edges at each end of the handle have to be sharpened.

Sickle scalers are universal instruments and, like universal curets, they are available with a straight or angulated shank.

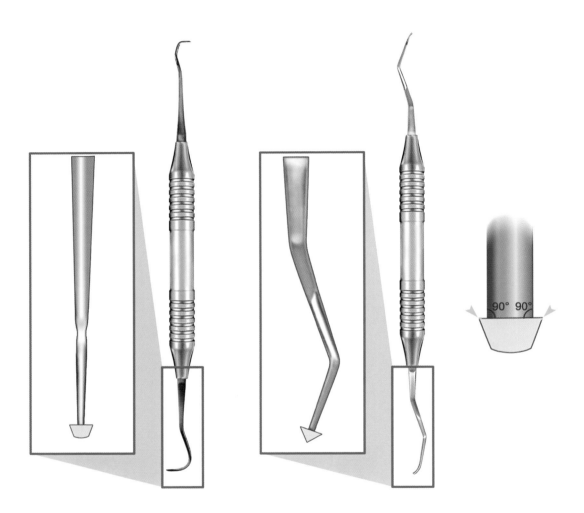

The face of the blade is at a right angle to the lower shank on both angulated- and straight-shanked scalers. Please note how the position of the handle will significantly vary among instruments so as to maintain the 20-degree angle between the stone and the lower part of instrument shank, as well as the correct 110 degree angle between the face of the blade and the stone, as illustrated in the following figure.

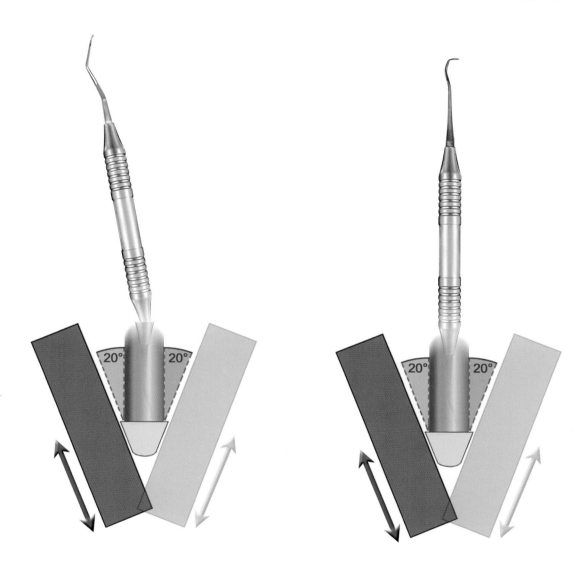

Sharpening a scaler with an angulated shank is more difficult than sharpening one with a straight shank, when using the stationary instrument/moving stone technique.

Therefore the stationary stone/moving instrument technique is especially recommended for sharpening scalers with angulated shanks.

Stationary stone/moving instrument technique

The 20-degree angle between the lower shank and the stone is also maintained in this sharpening technique, as shown in the following figures.

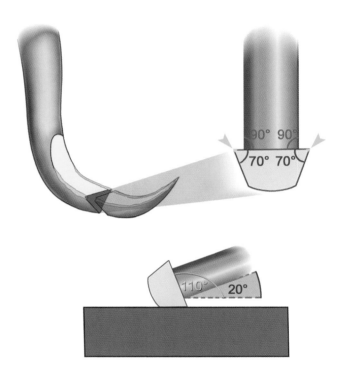

Both cutting edges at each end of the handle must be sharpened.

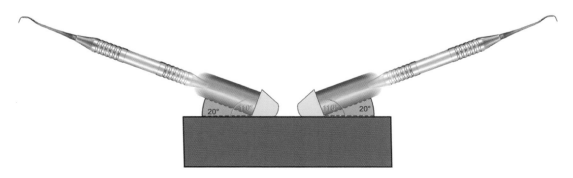

The stone is positioned on a stable working surface and a 20-degree angle between the stone and the lower shank must be created. To facilitate the procedure, a useful suggestion is to place the stone overhanging on the edge of the working surface, so that the lower part of the shank is initially laid down on the short side of the stone and immediately after slightly lifted,, as shown in the following figures, to maintain the correct 20-degrees angle, between the stone and the instrument lower shank.

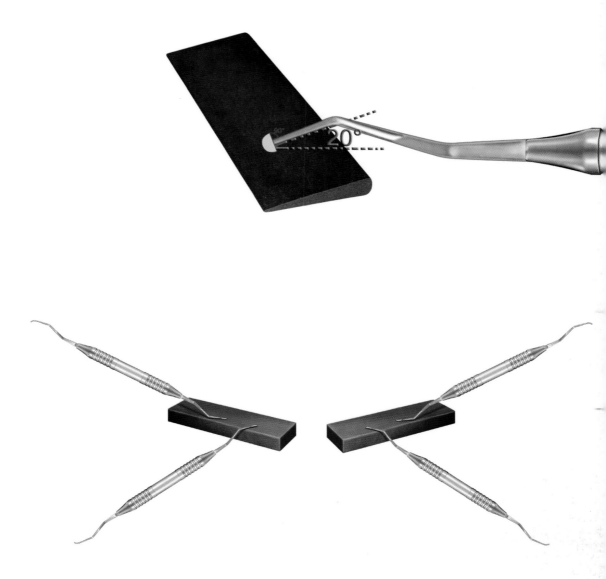

SHARPENING ANGLES TO REMEMBER

45°   Sharpening angle for the tip of all curets

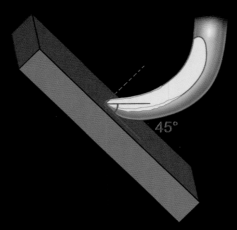

45°

40°   Sharpening angle for all area-specific curets

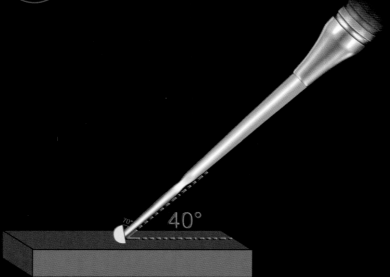

40°

Sharpening angle for all scalers

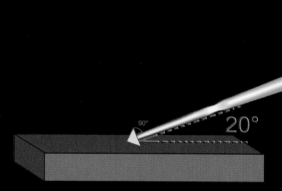

 Sharpening angle for all universal curets

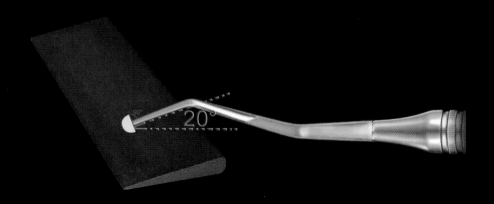

REFERENCES

1. Wilkins EM. Clinical Practice of the Dental Hygienist, ed 8. Philadelphia: Lippincott, William & Wilkins, 1999.

2. Benfenati MP, Montesani MT, Benfenati SP, Nathanson D. Scanning electron microscope: An SEM study of periodontally instrumented root surfaces, comparing sharp, dull, and damaged curettes and ultrasonic instruments. Int J Periodontics Restorative Dent 1987;7(2):50-67.

3. Silva MV, Gomes DA, Leite FR, Sampaio JE, de Toledo BE, Mendes AJ. Sharpening of periodontal instruments with different sharpening stones and its influence upon root debridement–scanning electronic microscopy assessment. J Int Acad Periodontol 2006;8(1):17-22.

4. Tal H, Kozlovsky A, Green E, Gabbay M. Scanning electron microscope evaluation of wear of stainless steel and high carbon steel curettes. J Periodontol 1989;60:320-4.

5. Checchi L, Pelliccioni GA, Trombelli L. Sharpening technics for periodontal instruments [in Italian]. Prev Assist Dent 1990;16(4):17-21.

6. Pattison AM, Pattison GL. Periodontal Instrumentation: Clinical Manual. Norwalk, CT: Appleton & Lange, 1992.

7. Pattison G, Pattison AM. Periodontal Instrumentation, ed 2. Upper Saddle River, NJ: Prentice Hall, 1992.

8. Moses O, Tal H, Artzi Z, Sperling A, Zohar R, Nemcovsky CE. Scanning electron microscope evaluation of two methods of resharpening periodontal curets: A comparative study. J Periodontol 2003;74:1032-1037.

9. Rossi R, Smukler H. A scanning electron microscope study comparing the effectiveness of different types of sharpening stones and curets. J Periodontol 1995;66:956-961.

10. Bash VC. An aid in sharpening explorers. J Am Dent Assoc 2004;135:1434-1435.

11. Römhild L, Renggli HH, San Giorgi MD. Sharpening periodontal instruments with help of Periostar precision sharpening system [in German]. Quintessenz 1990;41:267-278.

12. Woodall I. Comprehensive dental hygiene care, ed 4. St. Louis: Mosby, 1993.

13. Schwartz M. The prevention and management of the broken curet. Compend Contin Educ Dent 1998;19:418-425, vi.

14. Roncati M, Marzola P. il Kit Minimalista. Milan: Acme, 2006.

15. Houseman GA, Nield-Gehrig JS. Fundamentals of Dental Hygiene Instrumentation. Philadelphia: Saunders, 1983.

16. Murray GH, Lubow RM, Mayhew RB, Summitt JB, Usseglio RJ. The effects of two sharpening methods on the strength of a periodontal scaling instrument. J Periodontol 1984;55:410-413.

VERIFICATION
QUESTIONS
AND ANSWERS

GET SHARP
NONSURGICAL PERIODONTAL INSTRUMENT SHARPENING

1 **When sharpening all curets and scalers, the angle between the stone and the face of the blade should be maintained at:**
a) 110 degrees
b) 45 degrees
c) 20 degrees
(refer to pg. 92-93)

2 **Does the sharpening angle between stone and handle remain fixed for all instruments?**
a) No, the position of the handle varies in relation to the stone, even when sharpening different Gracey curets, to maintain the 110-degree angle between the facial surface and the stone
b) Yes, it is a 45-degree angle
c) Yes, it is a 40-degree angle
(refer to pg. 108)

3 **When sharpening the curet toe, at what angle should the stone be placed to the tip for all curets?**
a) 40 degrees
b) 20 degrees
c) 45 degrees
(refer to pg. 116)

4 **What is the sharpening angle between the lower part of the shank and the stone for scalers with a straight shank?**
a) 40 degrees
b) 20 degrees
c) 45 degrees
(refer to pg. 97)

5 **What is the sharpening angle between the lower part of the shank and the stone for scalers with an angulated shank?**
a) 20 degrees, the same as for scalers with a straight shank
b) 40 degrees
c) 45 degrees
(refer to pg. 82, 113)

6 **What is the sharpening angle between the lower part of the shank and the stone for universal curets?**
a) 40 degrees
b) 20 degrees, the same as for scalers because both are universal instruments
c) 45 degrees
(refer to pg. 67, 96)

7 **Which is the sharpening angle between the lower part of the shank and the stone for area-specific curets?**
a) 20 degrees
b) 45 degrees
c) 40 degrees for all area-specific curets (1/2 to 17/18) and for Curvette-type curets
(refer to pg. 71, 95, 98)

8 **Which is the sharpening angle between the tip of a scaler and the stone?**
a) 45 degrees
b) 40 degrees
c) Never sharpen the tip of a scaler because it must remain tapered rather than rounded like a curet
(refer to pg. 97)

9 **Before sharpening an instrument, the stone should be lubricated?**
a) With mineral oil or with petroleum jelly
b) With extra virgin olive oil
c) It is not necessary to lubricate the stone
(refer to pg. 37)

10 **How it is possible to remove metal stains left on the stone after instrument sharpening?**
a) The instrument is first sterilized, then it is rubbed with alcohol
b) Orange solvent is used before washing the stone to erase metal discoloration; after that the stone is sealed in an autoclave bag and properly sterilized

c) It is not possible to remove the metal stains from the stone
(refer to pg. 26)

11 It is possible to sterilize sharpening stones?
a) They must be sterilized like any other dental instrument
b) They must not be sterilized, but they can be dipped in boiling oil
c) They can be cleaned with a disinfectant spray
(refer to pg. 23)

12 How frequently must periodontal instruments be sharpened?
a) It is convenient to sharpen periodontal instruments at the first sign of operative inefficiency, because it is easier to restore the cutting edge before the instrument is overly worn
b) Once a month
c) Three or four times per year
(refer to pg. 22)

13 Why it is necessary to sharpen a periodontal instrument?
a) Because a sharpened instrument facilitates more effective instrumentation, causes less fatigue for the operator, prevents accidental trauma to soft tissue, does not need to be grasped in a tiring manner, and improves the tactile sensitivity of the clinician
b) To decrease the patient's comfort
c) To increase the time of treatment and to burnish the calculus
(refer to pg. 12, 15-16)

14 What happens if unsharpened instruments are used?
a) They will always be well-controlled by the operator
b) The operator may risk losing control of the instrument, may take longer to complete treatment, and may burnish the calculus

c) The operator will tend to apply less pressure
(refer to pg. 16-17)

15 What is the purpose of sharpening?
a) To restore the cutting edge and to maintain the original design of the instrument
b) To rapidly use up the instruments
c) To jeopardize the healing of instrumented site
(refer to pg. 14)

16 Why perform manual sharpening?
a) To save the price of a mechanical sharpening device
b) Because manual sharpening is the most rapid way to restore the cutting edge of instrument blades while working chair-side
c) Because mounted stones allow too delicate sharpening
(refer to pg. 20)

17 Which materials are needed for sharpening?
a) A sharpening stone, lubricant, the instruments to be sharpened, a small acrylic test stick, and a magnifying instrument
b) A mechanical sharpener
c) A diamond or aluminum oxide stone
(refer to pg. 29)

18 Which are stones of natural origin?
a) The diamond and ceramic stones
b) Only the India stone
c) India and Arkansas stones are quarried from natural mineral deposits
(refer to pg. 30)

19 For what purpose is the cylindrical stone used?
a) To begin the process of sharpening periodontal instruments
b) To sharpen faster
c) To eliminate sludge of metal shavings
(refer to pg. 90)

20 Which degree of stone abrasiveness is most often indicated?
a) A medium-grain stone such as the India stone
b) Abrasive stones should not be used
c) The most abrasive stone available
(refer to pg. 33-34)

21 Are periodontal files sharpened with an India stone?
a) No, periodontal files are sharpened with a specialized file sharpener that must be purchased when using this type of instrument
b) Yes
c) Yes, along with the Arkansas stone
(refer to pg. 35)

22 What is meant by shank of an instrument?
a) The handle
b) The part that includes the cutting edge
c) The part from the handle to the working end, divided into upper and lower parts
(refer to pg. 44)

23 In this text, reference is always made to the angle created between the stone and:
a) The lower part of the shank
b) The upper part of the shank
c) The shank
(refer to pg. 44, 116-117)

24 Are all curets area-specific instruments?
a) Yes
b) No, some curets are universal instruments
c) Yes, they are called Curvettes
(refer to pg. 61)

25 Do sickle scalers always have a straight shank?
a) No, some scalers have an angulated shank
b) Yes
c) Yes, but they can be modified by sharpening
(refer to pg. 60)

26 Do universal curets always have an angulated shank?
a) Yes, except for the 5/6 Langer curet
b) No, they all have a straight shank
c) Yes
(refer to pg. 61, 64)

27 What is the total number of cutting edges on a universal instrument?
a) Two
b) One
c) Four, two at each end of the handle
(refer to pg. 61)

28 **What are the main differences between universal and area-specific instruments?**
a) There are no differences
b) Universal instruments are scalers, and area-specific instruments are not
c) Universal instruments have two cutting edges at each end of the handle, while area-specific instruments have only one cutting edge at each end. Area-specific instruments are used on specific surfaces, while the universal ones can be used on any surface of the oral cavity
(refer to pg. 61, 84)

29 **The cutting edge of an instrument is formed:**
a) By the facial surface and the lateral surface of the working end
b) Between two lateral surfaces
c) Between the back and the lateral surface
(refer to pg. 47-49)

30 **What does burnishing calculus mean?**
a) Performing an effective instrumentation
b) Performing the instrumentation with a longer working time
c) Removing only a superficial portion of calculus present, leaving residual calcified deposits that jeopardize the complete healing of the site
(refer to pg. 17, 55)

Answers:
1.a / 2.a / 3.c / 4.b / 5.a / 6.b / 7.c / 8.c / 9.a / 10.b / 11.a / 12.a / 13.a / 14.b / 15.a / 16.b / 17.a / 18.c / 19.c / 20.a / 21.a / 22.c / 23.a / 24.b / 25.a / 26.a / 27.c / 28.c / 29.a / 30.c